THE STREAM OF BECOMING: A STUDY OF MARTHA ROGERS'S THEORY

Barbara Sarter, PhD, RN, CS
University of Southern California
Department of Nursing

Pub. No. 15-2205

National League for Nursing • New York

ISBN 0-88737-390-9

Manufactured in the United States of America

**To Kumarji
and our Family of Friends
with its Healing Touch
of Evolutionary Spirit**

CONTENTS

ACKNOWLEDGMENTS

I would like to express my deep appreciation to Dr. Gean Mathwig, Dr. Ardis Swanson, and Professor James C. Carse, all of New York University, for their invaluable support in this endeavor. Special thanks are due to Dr. Martha E. Rogers, who was the source of inspiration for this book, and who was so generous with her time and thoughts. Finally, words cannot express all that I owe to Dr. Naomi Aschner and my family, without whose support this effort would not have borne fruit.

INTRODUCTION

PHILOSOPHY, THEORY, AND SCIENCE

The discipline of nursing is assuming a significant role in the human sciences. Nursing as an activity has always held an important—indeed, essential—place in human life; but nursing as a distinctive scientific discipline has developed only in this century, with major advances made in the last three decades. The struggle for recognition within the scientific community has been long and hard, and is by no means over.

Nursing's preoccupation with establishing itself as a science has led to an emphasis on the conduct of quantitatively designed research, an attempt to define variables in measurable terms and to provide statistical analyses of relationships among variables. Nursing models have also been developed that attempt to organize conceptions of nursing, research, educational curricula, and practice. These models show a wide variety of views about nursing and its phenomena of concern. They have, unfortunately, been particularly weak in serving as generators of research hypotheses. The casual observer, when apprehending the diversity of nursing models in use, may well wonder if there is any unifying perspective, any basic agreement among nursing theorists, as to the nature of nursing and its phenomena of concern.

1

These two flaws in the realm of nursing models—their lack of research productivity and their diversity of views—indicate that the basic foundational work of the discipline has yet to be accomplished. Nursing research shows an alarming absence of theoretical relevance, and nursing theory displays wide divergence, because the profession has neglected the development and articulation of a philosophy of nursing. In a sense, our knowledge development has proceeded backwards—we have been attempting to conduct our science without first defining the fundamental perspective from which we approach reality, the methods of knowing we believe to be appropriate to that perspective, and the values inherent in it.

Such is the task of philosophy. The major branches of philosophical endeavor are metaphysics, epistemology, ethics, logic, and aesthetics. The first three of these correspond, respectively, to the above-mentioned activities. Metaphysics is the study of the essential nature of reality, epistemology the study of how we can know that reality, and ethics the study of how we should relate to it. Traditionally, philosophers have believed that the most fundamental of these branches is metaphysics. Two of the areas of concern to the metaphysician are ontology and teleology. Ontology deals with the nature of the real in its essence; that is, in abstraction from its specific manifestations. Teleology is the study of the goals, purposes, or values inherent in the universe. Ontological and teleological questions form the foundation a discipline's worldview, its overall perspective on life. These fundamental issues must be dealt with before the concerns of epistemology and ethics can be satisfactorily addressed. The present work is an effort to establish the ontological and teleological foundations of the discipline of nursing.

In recent years, a number of nursing scholars have called for just such a "foundational analysis."[1] Donaldson and Crowley were among the first. In their landmark article, "The Discipline of Nursing," they held up a standard by which to measure the status of nursing as a discipline: "A discipline is characterized by a unique perspective, a distinct way of viewing all phenomena, which ultimately defines the limits and nature of its reality."[2] More recently, such eminent theorists as Leininger[3] and Watson have specifically identified ontological and teleological issues as being of central import to the discipline. Watson is one of the few nursing theorists to actually have identified her work as directed toward the establishment of a metaphysical context for nursing. In her most recent book, she identified the problem in this way: "Nursing still has a long way to go in adopting a meaningful philosophical foundation for its theories and its science that is consistent with past and present visions, images, and ideals of nursing leaders."[4]

Scholars in nursing are now realizing that the identification of a philosophical foundation for nursing is, ideally, a precondition for theory development and productive research. Science and philosophy, however, exist in a mutually complementary relationship. A philosophy that is unaware of or ignores scientific information is in danger of being inaccurate or, worse, completely untrue. A science that lacks any larger perspective than what it records from one research project to another is in danger of becoming lost in an ocean of detail. Additionally, current philosophers of science maintain that all fact is "theory-laden," in the sense that the mind always influences perception. It becomes particularly important, then, to clarify our basic assumptions about the world.

Much discussion in recent years has revolved around the importance of a "metaparadigm" for the discipline of nursing. A metaparadigm is described in various terms, but the essence of the concept is that it is the fundamental worldview agreed upon by all members of the discipline. The metaparadigm defines what concepts are significant to the field, identifies the point of view to be taken when studying the phenomena of interest to the discipline, and outlines the appropriate methodologies to be used in researching these phenomena. Clearly, the metaparadigm of a discipline will flow directly from the philosophical assumptions the discipline embraces. In other words, the underlying philosophical assumptions of a discipline *are* its metaparadigm.

The concepts of person, environment, health/illness, and nursing have been accepted as the backbone of a metaparadigm for nursing. Indeed, Fawcett has maintained that these four concepts alone constitute nursing's metaparadigm.[5] But a mere statement of concepts does not form a complete metaparadigm. These concepts may form the framework for a metaparadigm, but identifying them is only the first step. It is true that all of nursing's conceptual models and theories deal with one or more of these concepts. A wide divergence of approaches to and definitions of these concepts is seen, however, and often the viewpoints are virtually incompatible. For example, a definition of person as a unitary four-dimensional energy field is radically different from a definition of person as a set of behavioral subsystems. The metaphysical, epistemological, and ethical implications of each of these views are likewise in conflict.

Although there is nearly universal agreement within the discipline that a plurality of nursing models and theories is desirable, it is another issue entirely as to whether a plurality of metaparadigms is possible without losing the status of a discipline. According to Donaldson and Crowley's definition, a *unified* perspective, or worldview, is necessary in order to claim the status of a discipline. Can we agree on any characteristics of a metaparadigm for nursing besides a few named concepts? In order to achieve consensus on a metaparadigm, nursing theorists must be willing to acknowledge their fundamental similarities of perspective and also, perhaps, to sacrifice some of their individual differences.

Significant statements have been made by several nursing scholars regarding the general themes and subject matter that should be included in a metaparadigm for nursing. Donaldson and Crowley identify the thematic boundaries for the discipline of nursing as follows: (1) the principles and laws governing human life-processes and well-being; (2) the patterning of human/environment interaction in critical life situations; and (3) the processes by which positive changes in health status are affected.[6] More recently, Watson was quite specific in describing a human science context for nursing. She identifies the following philosophical commitments:

- Human beings are nonreducible experiencing subjects characterized by freedom, choice, and responsibility.

- There is an interconnected evolution of the human and the world; nurse and person are coparticipants in ongoing change.

- Health is a process.

- An epistemology for nursing should allow for aesthetics, ethics, intuition, and process discovery.[7]

Perhaps the most fundamental question that needs to be answered in order to develop nursing's metaparadigm is, What is the nature of the human being? Our answer to this question will determine, in turn, how we view human health and illness, human/environment interaction, and the nurse/patient relationship.

The philosophical discussion in the following pages presents one effort to answer this question. The science of unitary human beings, the most abstract and philosophically complex of nursing's conceptual frameworks, provides an excellent focus for philosophical analysis. This model has also had a profound influence on the discipline as a whole. Many of its basic concepts have stimulated fruitful theory development, research, and practice. One may safely say that without Rogers's pioneering effort to bring the revolutions of physics and biology into the arena of nursing knowledge, the discipline would be at a very different point in its development. A clarification, then, of the metaphysical implications of Rogers's model and suggestions for strengthening its philosophical coherence will contribute to the metaparadigm development of the entire discipline.

THE METHOD OF PHILOSOPHICAL RESEARCH

Philosophical research and philosophy are not the same activity. Philosophy forms the subject matter for philosophical research. One goal of philosophical research, however, may be to generate new philosophy. Thus, two questions must be answered: What is philosophy, and what is philosophical research?

Simply defined, philosophy is inquiry into the nature of reality through rational or intuitive thought. The traditional goal of philosophy is wisdom, or an understanding of truth. Philosophical research is the investigation of selected works of philosophy for the purpose of answering a specific philosophical question or problem. Through the process of philosophical research, the researcher comes to understand how others have approached similar or related problems, evaluates the validity of various philosophers' answers, and, if possible or necessary, develops new insights or solutions.

When a discipline other than philosophy engages in philosophical research, the research question must be framed within a context of meaning to that discipline. This is known as applied philosophy. As suggested in our earlier discussion of the nature of a discipline, one can say that all disciplines must have a philosophy, whether implicit or explicit. A distinction may be made between philosophy *for* a discipline and the philosophy *of* a discipline. The former is the use of ideas or methods from philosophy to aid in the work of a discipline. To develop a philosophy of nursing, however, is to create a new and unique perspective on the discipline's phenomena of interest. For example, the methods of positivistic philosophy have been utilized essentially unchanged to create and evaluate nursing research. Positivism has been used *for* nursing. The task of nursing philosophers is to articulate a unique philosophy *of* nursing.

The approaches that are possible for philosophical research are numerous. One may choose a historical approach. One may choose to focus on only the "giants" among philosophers. One may choose to research only contemporary thought on a problem. These are structurally relatively simple approaches. The framework for research may take a more complex form, however. For example, it may take a dialectical form. The essential components of a dialectic are thesis, antithesis, and synthesis. By examining opposite points of view on the problem under investigation, the researcher attempts to find a perspective of balance between the two extremes. The synthesis is not actually a middle point, but rather a unique and more complex product, which, ideally achieves a higher level of knowledge than the thesis or antithesis. Another approach is to illuminate or clarify a set of ideas by comparing them to others' ideas dealing with the same content area. There are many other possible approaches to philosophical research. As in other forms of research, the problem chosen for investigation should be the determinant of the method to be used.

EVALUATING PHILOSOPHY

In traditional empirical research, the "truth" of a hypothesis is tested by statistical analysis. How is the truth of a philosophical idea or system evaluated? Several approaches to determining the truth of a philosophy have been utilized throughout the centuries. One of the most commonly used standards is the explanatory power of a philosophy. How much of the vast range of human experience does it satisfactorily explain? A closely related criterion is the comprehensiveness of the philosophy. Does it take into account all possible factors relevant to the topic of study? Another criterion of truth is coherence. Do all the parts of the system of ideas fit together logically? Do the individual elements reflect the overall meaning of the system? Aesthetic criteria have also been used. Does the philosophy demonstrate qualities such as elegance and simplicity? The American pragmatist school of philosophy identified yet another approach to defining truth. Their approach was that any idea that proves to be useful in the "real world" or that creates consensus among a community of scholars may be called true.[8]

Another important approach to evaluating the truth of a philosophy developed out of the scientific approach to knowledge development. The empiricist school of philosophy, expressed most brilliantly in the works of Bertrand Russell, established a set of correspondence criteria of truth. The philosopher or theorist is expected to establish the closest possible correspondence between his ideas and factual reality. Factual reality refers to a reality that is objective, perceivable by all, and verifiable.

The theories of truth described above reflect various epistemological views. It is not difficult to see that the epistemological approach used implies a certain set of underlying metaphysical assumptions. For example, the epistemology of correspondence is based on the metaphysical view known as materialism. The discipline of nursing, which for decades has accepted the correspondence view of truth in evaluating its research, has recently begun to question the metaphysic of materialism on which it is based.

The intuitionist school of philosophy has identified yet another way of evaluating the truth of a philosophy or theory. Polanyi and others from this school maintain that personal intuition is the most compelling criterion of truth.[9] Even when other criteria, such as any of those mentioned above, are ostensibly in use, the ultimate and final judge of truth is the intuition of the evaluator. The intuitionists have used the term "theory-laden fact" to capture the idea that there is no such thing as pure fact. The mind-set of the observer is always influencing perception.

EVALUATING PHILOSOPHICAL RESEARCH

Since the goal of philosophical research is not always to develop a new philosophy, other criteria may be necessary for evaluating it. Of course, if the researcher has set out to propose a new philosophical view, then any of the criteria described above may be used. The starting point is always the research question. Is the question significant? Is the method proposed to answer the question or problem appropriate? Is the method actually utilized congruent with the method that was proposed? Are the primary sources of philosophy to be examined suitable for the research question? Is the interpretation and analysis of primary sources accurate? Are the conclusions of the researcher logically developed and clearly stated? Is the knowledge or perspective gained by the research of significance to the discipline? Does it contribute to the development of the philosophical foundations of the discipline? These are some of the major points that can be used to assist in the evaluation of a piece of philosophical research.

PLANNING A PHILOSOPHICAL RESEARCH PROJECT

The above discussion of philosophical research was intended, in part, to serve as an introduction to the work presented in the following pages. To date, only a small number of philosophical studies have been conducted within the discipline of nursing. Thus, any study of this type that is presented to the profession carries with it the responsibility of serving as a model and precedent. It may be helpful to the reader to be provided with some details about the development of this particular study.

As is true of most research projects, the initial formulation took a general and broad form. Because of the prominence of the concepts of evolution and holism in Rogers's model, these were recognized as important areas for philosophical analysis. It seemed clear that Rogers was using these old ideas in a very new way. It also was clear that many students of the model of unitary human beings had some difficulty in understanding or accepting Rogers's view of the person and of evolution. Finally, a number of philosophers have attempted to deal with these issues throughout the ages. It appeared that an examination of how some of the great thinkers of the world had described holistic human beings and evolution might help to clarify Rogerian theory.

Moving from a broad area of interest and significance to a specific and researchable problem statement is perhaps the most difficult step in any type of research activity. In philosophical research, one of the first decisions to be made is what branch of philosophy is most appropriate to frame the research question and guide the investigation. Is the area of interest most suitable to an epistemological, metaphysical, ethical, logical, or aesthetic mode of inquiry? Although a given content area may be approached from more than one field, usually one branch of philosophy will show a particular suitability for handling the issues. Metaphysics was determined to be the most appropriate form of inquiry for this area of inquiry.

Metaphysics is the study of the most basic characteristics and problems of existence. Reason, intuition, and experience have been identified as the tools of metaphysics, which is felt by many to be the foundation stone of philosophy. Aristotle described metaphysics as the science of "first principles." Taylor has set forth some of the questions with which the metaphysician deals:

What am I? What is this world, and why is it such? Why is it not like the moon—
bleak, barren, hostile, meaningless? How can such a thing as this be? What is
this brain?; does it think? And this craving or will, whence does it arise? Is it
free? Does it perish with me, or not? Is it perhaps everlasting? What is death?
And life—is it a clockwork? Does the world offer no alternatives? And if so, does
it matter? What can one think about the gods, if anything at all? Are there any?
Or is nature herself her own creator, and the creator of me; both cradle and tomb,
both holy and mundane, both heaven and hell?[10]

One can see that although Rogers would vigorously deny that she is a
metaphysician, she has attempted to deal with some of these questions in
her model. That is why the model is considered to be the most abstract and
complex of our discipline. Examining the metaphysical implications of
Rogers's conceptualizations seemed a highly significant task to pursue. But
again, the researcher's perpetual problem presented itself. Neither the model
in its entirety nor the field of metaphysical analysis in its entirety could be
taken on, appealing as that might have been. The area of focus needed to
be narrowed. I decided to examine two specific concepts within the model
that presented some basic metaphysical problems: (1) the human energy field
and (2) the principle of helicy. I felt the former was the fundamental ontological unit of Rogers's worldview. The latter addressed some teleological
problems associated with the concept of evolution. Some further explanation of the terms ontology and teleology may be helpful.

As mentioned earlier, ontology is concerned with the nature of reality in
its essence, in abstraction from its specific manifestations. It is also known
as the philosophy of being. Ontology attempts to answer one basic question:
What is real? Through the writings of selected philosophers, this study explored the specific question: What is the nature of the human being? Rogers's
concept of the human energy field was felt to represent the ontological implications of the model.

Teleology is the attempt by metaphysicians to discover the goals, purposes,
or values inherent in the universe. Traditionally, teleological causation has
been characterized as involving a mental will or purpose, an end result, that
influences natural processes in the present. The more modern use of the word
refers simply to purposive or goal-oriented processes. The specific teleological
question explored in this study was, What is the goal or purpose of human
evolution? Rogers's principle of helicy was selected as most revealing of the
teleological implications of the model.

Thus, the broad area of metaphysics was narrowed down to the areas of
ontology and teleology. In turn, the ontology of human beings and the
teleology of evolution were selected as being most appropriate for a study
of relevance to nursing theory. Finally, two specific concepts from Rogers's
model were selected as being the most fruitful foci for clarifying some of
the metaphysical implications of the discipline of nursing.

Further issues remained to be resolved before the research could proceed systematically. The methodological options discussed above were weighed, and a combination of approaches was decided upon: a historical approach, presumably, a modified dialectical form for the main substance of the study; and an in-depth analysis of the opposite views of materialism and idealism, with the purpose of establishing a spectrum of thought against which Rogers's ontological and teleological implications could be illuminated. Two modern philosophers were selected as representatives of each of these views—Jacques Monod for the materialist view, and Pierre Teilhard de Chardin for the idealist view. Selected writings of each of these philosophers were analyzed and critiqued. A synthesis of the materialist and idealist views was not sought. It was possible that Rogers's model would be revealed as being such a synthesis, however. This would not be known until the research process was completed.

The final task of planning the research was to decide what the ultimate goal of the study would be. Would it be a comparison and contrast? Would it be only to identify the metaphysical implications of the model? Because the ultimate purpose of philosophical research is theory development, not only theory analysis, the first two options were not satisfactory. It would be preferable to *evaluate* the metaphysical implications uncovered and, if problems emerged, to *suggest* how the model might be made philosophically more solid. Thus, the last decision to be made was what criterion would be used to evaluate the model's ontological and teleological implications. The decision was made to use the criterion of coherence, as described by Joachim.[11]

To summarize the narrowing-down and focusing process that was involved in the planning of this research, the first step was to identify what branch of philosophy would be most appropriate for exploring the area of interest. Next, a decision had to be made as to what particular philosophical issues and what particular elements of the model would be clarified and analyzed in depth. Choosing a method that would yield the richest possible results was the next major decision. Selecting the particular philosophers and choosing the particular primary sources for intensive study was of critical importance. It may be mentioned here that in addition to using Rogers's written works, the researcher also conducted personal interviews with her. This added to the richness of information available about the model. Finally, the goals and desired outcomes of the research needed to be detailed, and evaluation criteria specified.

The result of planning the research was the identification of six specific research questions or problems statements:

1. What are the ontological implications of Rogers's view of evolution as reflected in her conception of the human energy field?

2. What are the teleological implications of Rogers's view of evolution as reflected in the principle of helicy?

3. What is the overall metaphysical theme of Rogers's view of evolution?

4. Is Rogers's implied ontology coherent in relation to the overall metaphysical theme of her model?

5. Is Rogers's implied teleology coherent in relation to the overall metaphysical theme of her model?

6. What changes, if any, are needed in Rogers's model to enhance the systematic coherence of her metaphysic?

In addition to answering these research questions, I identified the following insights and understandings as goals of the research:

1. An understanding of two metaphysical issues involved in the development of an evolutionary view of man—ontology and teleology

2. An understanding of how these issues have been dealt with by philosophers of the past and by two modern philosophers

3. A critical analysis of some central concepts of Rogers's model of unitary human beings that deal with the ontology and teleology of evolution

4. An evaluation of these metaphysical implications of Rogers's model according to their coherence with the overalll metaphysical theme of the model

5. Suggestions for further elaboration of a metaphysically coherent evolutionary nursing philosophy that can be used as a basis for the development of holistic nursing theory.

The following chapters will present the substance of this philosophical research. The intellectual steps will be presented in logical sequence so that the reader's understanding will be taken from the general to the specific. First, a historical overview of evolutionary philosophy will be presented. The opposing metaphysical views of materialism and idealism will be analyzed and critiqued primarily through the examination of two modern philosophers, with reference to others as well. At the conclusion of the presentation of this background work, the reader will have an understanding of the ontological and teleological stances traditionally associated with the materialistic and idealistic views of evolution. Next, Rogers's model will be described, analyzed in relation to the metaphysical spectrum previously established, and evaluated for its systematic coherence. Suggestions will then be offered as to how the metaphysical foundations of this model and of nursing theory as a whole may be strengthened and made more coherent and more reflective of nursing's commitment to holistic and humanistic care. The transcripts of the interviews conducted with Dr. Rogers as part of the data collection are included in the appendix.

It should be emphasized, finally, that a philosophical study such as this must be read in sequence. The logic of the analytical process demands this. The reader should try to resist the temptation to jump ahead to the final chapter to gain a "sneak preview" of the conclusions drawn. Proceed with patience, and cover with me every step of the journey!

REFERENCES

1. Paula Manchester, "Analytic Philosophy and Foundational Inquiry: The Method," in *Nursing Research: A Qualitative Perspective,* ed. P. L. Munhall and P. Oiler (Norwalk, CT: Appleton-Century-Crofts, 1986).

2. S. K. Donaldson and D. M. Crowley, "The Discipline of Nursing," *Nursing Outlook,* 26 (1978), 113–20.

3. Madeleine M. Leininger, "Nature, Rationale, and Importance of Qualitative Research Methods in Nursing," in *Qualitative Research Methods in Nursing,* ed. M. M. Leininger (Orlando, FL: Grune & Stratton, 1985).

4. Jean Watson, *Nursing: Human Science and Human Care* (Norwalk, CT: Appleton-Century-Crofts, 1985), p. 78.

5. Jacqueline Fawcett, *Analysis and Evaluation of Conceptual Models of Nursing* (Philadelphia: F. A. Davis, 1984).

6. Donaldson and Crowley, "The Discipline of Nursing."

7. Watson, *Nursing,* p. 16.

8. L. Armour, *The Concept of Truth* (Assen: Van Gorcum and Company, 1969).

9. Michael Polanyi, *Personal Knowledge* (London: Routledge & Kegan Paul, 1958).

10. Richard Taylor, *Metaphysics* (Englewood Cliffs, NJ: Prentice-Hall, 1974), p. 7.

11. Harold H. Joachim, "Truth as Coherence," in *Contemporary Philosophic Problems,* ed. Y. H. Krikorian and A. Edel (New York: Macmillan, 1959).

2

VIEWS OF THE BECOMING: PHILOSOPHICAL SPECULATIONS ANCIENT AND MODERN

The constant search for a deeper understanding of life and the universe in which it exists has been the wellspring of philosophical inquiry throughout the ages. Every generation seems to feel the need to reask and reanswer questions about the nature, meaning, and purpose of our world. It is foolish to believe that those who lived in other times and cultures cannot provide the current age with any perspectives of relevance. From the time the Aryan sages recorded the Vedas several thousand years ago, virtually all possible metaphysical and epistemological views have been set forth. Thus, it is important that contemporary thinkers explore the wisdom and insights of those in previous ages in order to gain the widest possible perspective on their own philosophical concerns.

Within the discipline of nursing, some fundamental philosophical questions are concerned with the nature of human beings, the nature of the environment, and the relationship between the two. Conceptions of health, illness, and nursing will be derived from the positions taken on these issues. Nursing's as yet ill-defined position can be characterized by three general descriptors: holistic, evolutionary, and humanistic. In turning to the vast body of philosophical exposition from the time of classical Greece to the present, this chapter will highlight those thinkers who focused on the "stream of becoming"—the continuous flow of change in the world—and the nature of human evolution within this stream. The historical review will provide a background for the contrast of two contemporary expressions of materialism and idealism. This metaphysical background and spectrum of contemporary stances will provide a point of reference for the ultimate goal of this book— the clarification and strengthening of a metaphysical foundation for nursing science.

PRE-SOCRATICS[1]

The roots of both materialism and idealism in Western philosophy are found in early Greek thought. The pre-Socratic philosophers (ca. 600 B.C.), particularly the Ionics (Thales, Anaximander, and Anaximenes), conceive the basic substance of the world to consist of various perceptible elements. They do not look beyond the world of the senses. Thus they can be considered the fathers of scientific materialism. Thales believes that the primary substance of the world is water; Anaximander holds it to be a boundless, indefinite substance; and Anaximenes claims that it is vapor or air. Anaximander's view of evolution is that living creatures arose from water, and that man was born from the fishes.

Heraclitus (ca. 500 B.C.) and Empedocles (b. 490 B.C.) introduce the more subtle conceptualization of forces that underlie the perpetual flux of the world. For Heraclitus, the basic substance of the world is fire, which is also described as life, reason, and soul. Inherent in this world-stuff is an orderliness of transformation that directs the world's becoming. Empedocles assumes a pluralistic view of the world-substance, describing the four elements of earth, air, fire, and water as being mixed and molded by the forces of love and strife to create the evolution of living beings. First, plants arose from a primitive organic compound; the the evolution of animals and man followed. Those forms that survived were suited to their environment.

The atomism of Democritus (b. 460 B.C.) and Epicurus (b. 342 B.C.) became a cornerstone of modern scientific materialism. Both philosophers see the world as composed of invisible units of inert matter, indivisible and eternal. All the variety of the world is attributable to random collisions and combinations of these units. All change is mechanistic in character, caused by the motions of these atoms in empty space. For Epicurus, life and its evolution is a result of random swerves or variations in the paths of these atoms.

Anaxagoras (b. 500 B.C.) was the first Western philosopher to formulate a distinction between mind and matter, and also the first to introduce a teleological view of nature's becoming. Anaxagoras conceives the moving force of the world-process as being nonphysical, incorporeal. This force is called Nous—mind, intelligence. Here and in Heraclitus is the first attempt to introduce a principle of reason into the natural world. Plato and Aristotle further develop this germinal idea into full-scale idealistic systems.

PLATO AND ARISTOTLE[2]

The World-Soul of Plato (b. 427 B.C.) is a principle of animation that transforms the random movement of matter into purposive, living activity. The world of Forms, or Ideas, generates the world Becoming by infusing Matter with Soul. Forms are the universal, unchanging, eternal realities that are the essence of the visible world of becoming. Aristotle (b. 384 B.C.) places Plato's Forms within the structure of Matter, postulating an "entelechy," which is the "final cause" of an object's or organism's self-realization. The potentiality of Matter becomes actualized in part by the influence of Form, which is, itself, pure Actuality.

Aristotle's doctrine of causality has provided a basis for philosophical discussion among all subsequent generations. In this doctrine is found the first explication of teleological causation. For Aristotle, a complete explanation of the world-order must include four types of causation. There is, first of all, the material cause of a thing, the Matter itself. Second, there is the Form, or formal cause, which directs the development of a thing. This may be either an internal tendency of growth or an idea within the mind of an artificer. Third, the efficient cause is the agent or precedent whose initial action begins the process of development. Last, there is the end result, or goal, which is implicit as a potential in the object as it develops. This last form of causation is the traditional basis for teleological explanation.

NEO-PLATONISM[3]

The Neo-Platonic tradition, established by Plotinus in the second century A.D., provides a synthesis of Platonism and Aristotelianism in a monistic idealism. Plotinus's doctrine of emanation views the physical world as an outpouring or extension of divinity, the One. Plotinus denies a separate ontological status to matter, but does not deny the reality and integrity of individual beings, which are nonetheless parts of the immanent, yet transcendent, One. Like the World-Soul of Plato, Plotinus's world-soul serves a mediative role between mind and matter.

Giordano Bruno (b. 1548) combines a mechanistic view of causation with a Neo-Platonic teleology. Bruno conceives organisms as being composed of monads, which are at once corporeal and soul-like, eternal and mirroring the All. The Absolute is the primal unity, from which the world unfolds and which serves as the inner guiding principle of motion in nature. The combinations of monads are in constant change; only after repeated trials do species become adaptable and stable. Here can be seen the randomness of mechanistic motion occuring within a teleological substratum. The basic substance, consisting of monads, is essentially soul-like in nature.

RATIONALISM[4]

The 17th-century rationalists Descartes, Spinoza, and Leibniz provide distinctive variations of one basic theme, the primacy of reason in providing true knowledge of the world. René Descartes (b. 1596), considered by many the father of modern philosophy, established an ontological dualism of mind and matter that persists into the present day. Nature is totally devoid of consciousness, consisting only of matter in mechanical motion. The essence of matter is extension. Only the human mind, separate from the human body, is characterized by consciousness. All change in nature is explainable by purely deterministic mechanisms; teleology has no place whatever in natural processes.

Spinoza (b. 1632), in his absolute monism, sees mind and matter as two aspects of the one, all-embracing, divine substance. God is substance, as well as nature. Spinoza's monism is accompanied by a strict determinism: All events in nature flow of necessity from the divine nature. Since there is no interaction between mind and matter, teleology is emphatically rejected. However, Spinoza proposes that the human mind follows a process of development from imagination, through reason, to a scientific intuition in which one can identify with the infinite intellect of God. Bodies, too, form a hierarchy according to the complexity of their structure and function. Furthermore, each thing strives to complete its perfection of being, its essence, which is ultimately its relatedness to the whole. In this sense, then, Harris points out, "The ultimate explanation of things in Spinoza's system is teleological."[5]

The philosophy of Leibniz (b. 1646) attempts to synthesize teleology and mechanism. Force is the underlying substance of reality and takes the form of metaphysical atoms called monads. These simple, irreducible units contain a vital principle, or entelechy, endowed with the faculty of perception and with a plurality of affections and relations. Monads are distinguished from each other by the clarity of their perceptions. Because space, itself, is only a pattern of perceptions, monads are not "in space"; hence, they are windowless, in no spatial relation with each other. All change occurring in nature is due to a preestablished harmony among the monads. The nature of each monad is to strive for the full realization of its potentiality, which is ultimately to enter into the mind of God in complete clarity of perception. This inner impulse provides a teleological substratum for all physical laws.

GERMAN IDEALISM[6]

The triad of German idealists—Fichte, Schelling, and Hegel—all hold similar cosmological philosophies. Consciousness is seen as the active principle of the universe, the Absolute having become nature in order to realize itself as self-conscious spirit. Hegel (b. 1770) views the Becoming as a process of evolving self-consciousness. All natural processes of change and development are particular cases of the fundamental dialectical principle of unity in difference. The moving force of Becoming is the whole, immanent in each part and each moment of reality, urging every existent toward greater completion and wholeness. Like Leibniz, Hegel reconciles efficient and final causation by viewing mechanistic events as manifestations of a teleological world-process.

POST-DARWINIAN PHILOSOPHIES[7]

Darwin's landmark *Origin of Species,* published in 1864, had the effect of shifting the philosophical view of evolution as a logical process to a view of it as a temporal process. It also, through the theory of natural selection, provided a mechanistic explanation of the evolutionary process, dispensing with all concepts of purpose. Evolution occurs through the differential reproduction of mutant organisms: those mutants that are most adaptive to the changing environment of the species survive and proliferate. By no means, however, was the debate between materialism and idealism over. Indeed, the view of evolution as a process in time inspired several philosophers to break out of the restrictive, static monism of Spinoza and Hegel, into dynamic, process-oriented idealistic systems. The philosophies of Bergson and Whitehead are perhaps the most brilliant of the post-Darwinian idealisms. Spencer, Alexander, Smuts, Morgan, and Sellars proposed highly innovative evolutionary interpretations within the materialistic philosophical tradition.

Herbert Spencer (b. 1820) actually developed his materialistic philosophy of evolution prior to the publication of Darwin's exposition of natural selection. Spencer sees the entire universe as an eternal, continuous succession of cycles involving three stages—Evolution, Equilibration, and Dissolution. The ultimate ontology of the universe is unknowable; however, Force is the underlying principle of the knowable universe. Spencer's cosmic Law of Evolution delineates the direction of the process as being toward increasing complexity, integration, and diversification.

In the early 20th century, Samuel Alexander, J.C. Smuts, and C. Lloyd Morgan held essentially materialistic views of "evolutionary emergence," a term initially used by Morgan. Emergence implies a creative advance of nature in which qualitatively new and unpredictable properties unfold as the complexity of form increases. In this way, the underlying continuity of substance allows a monistic ontology of the universe, while at the same time the emergence of new levels of existence, such as life and mind, can be explained. Alexander's ontology posits the universe to be grounded in Space-Time or Motion, whereas for Smuts it is grounded in Energy. Smuts develops the concept of holism in his philosophy, describing evolution as the development of increasingly integrated wholes. Morgan, alone of the three early emergent evolutionists, assumes a teleological impulse underlying the world-process.

Roy Wood Sellars (b. 1880) elegantly developed his critical evolutionary naturalism in a manner similar to that of the early emergentists. He, too, maintains that matter evolves into hierarchical levels of organization in which new properties and degrees of freedom emerge. Sellars's ontology is a pluralistic materialism revised to incorporate the modern view of evolution. Rather than being inert and characterized only by extension, matter is described as being dynamic, relational, and self-organizing.

Henri Bergson was one of the most widely acclaimed philosophers of evolution in the early 20th century. His *Creative Evolution* (1907) identifies reality as the élan vital, or vital flow, out of which matter emerges as a backward current. Life, creativity, change, and movement are innate in the élan, which flows into numerous divergent lines with complete freedom and spontaneity. Evolution involves no overall direction, being completely free and indeterminate. The mechanical appearance of the material world is a product of the human intellect, made to meet pragmatic needs. Evolution involves no overall direction, being the result of the indeterminacy, diversity, and liberty of the élan.

Alfred North Whitehead (b. 1861) refused to bifurcate nature into mind and matter. He rejects the notion of substance altogether and speaks of an enduring body as being a succession of "actual occasions." The basic elements of any actual occasion are prehensions, which involve emotion, purpose, valuation, and causation. Hence, actual occasions are "throbs of emotion," even at the atomic and molecular levels. Every actual occasion is a process of becoming, and once the satisfaction of its subjective aim is accomplished, the entity perishes and becomes a datum of prehension for other actual occasions. Whitehead's ontology is monistic but dipolar, in that every actual entity consists of a mental pole and a physical pole, which are inseparable and complementary. The evolutionary process is a development of feeling into increasing intensity, creativity, and novelty. An overall teleology of evolution is suggested in the final chapter of Whitehead's *Process and Reality,* where the Many are described as becoming One.

In this historical review of descriptions of the Becoming, certain themes and issues can be seen to have recurred throughout the ages. Ontological positions range from a perception of reality as purely matter to the view that only mind exists, and from monism to pluralism. Matter has been described as consisting of various physical elements, such as fire, water, atoms, or air. Idealists have identified more subtle spiritual or mental forces—such as reason, soul, vital energy, or consciousness—as the basic substance of the universe. Teleological explanations range from complete rejection of any purposiveness in the change inherent in the universe, to a view that the entire Becoming is goal-oriented. The goal itself has been variously depicted as complete freedom and creativity, Divinity, increasing complexity, or other fulfilled potentialities. In the following chapters, we will see many of these same ideas and themes interpreted and expressed by the philosophers Jacques Monod and Pierre Teilhard de Chardin. We will then turn to nursing theory to examine the ideas of our discipline against this backdrop, focusing primarily on Rogers, and briefly analyzing some other nursing theories for their philosophical implications.

REFERENCES

1. Resources used in relation to the pre-Socratics were John Burnett, *Early Greek Philosophy,* 4 ed. (London: Adam & Charles Black, 1930); B. A. G. Fuller, *A History of Philosophy,* 3 ed., rev. by Sterling M. McMurrin (New York: Henry Holt, 1955); William T. Stace, *A Critical History of Greek Philosophy* (London: Macmillan, 1920); Rex Warner, *The Greek Philosophers* (New York: New American Library, 1958).

2. Resources used in relation to Plato and Aristotle were Aristotle, *Selected Works,* trans. and ed. R. P. Hardie and R. K. Gaye (New York: Random House, 1941); Conrad Bonifazi, *The Soul of the World* (Washington: University Press of America, 1978); Burnett; Fuller; C. E. M. Joad, *Guide to Philosophy* (New York: Dover, 1936); Bertrand Russell, *A History of Western Philosophy* (New York: Simon and Schuster, 1945); Stace; Warner.

3. Resources used in relation to Neo-Platonism were Bonifazi; James C. Carse, *Death and Existence: A Conceptual History of Human Mortality* (New York: Wiley, 1980); Richard Falckenberg, *History of Modern Philosophy,* 3 ed., trans. A. C. Armstrong (Calcutta: Progressive Publishers, 1953); Fuller; Sarvepelli Radhakrishnan, ed., *History of Philosophy, Eastern and Western* (London: George Allen & Unwin, 1952); Warner.

4. Resources used in relation to rationalism were Bonifazi; Fuller; Errol E. Harris, *Nature, Mind and Modern Science* (London: George Allen & Unwin, 1954); Harold Hoffding, *A History of Modern Philosophy,* Vol I, trans. B. E. Meyer (rpt. New York: Dover, 1955); Gottfried W. Leibniz, *Selections,* ed. P. Wiener (New York: Scribner's, 1951); Russell; Benedict de Spinoza, *Ethics,* ed. James Gutmann (New York: Hafner, 1949).

5. Harris, *Nature, Mind and Modern Science,* p. 215.

6. Resources used in relation to German Idealism were Bonifazi; Fuller; Harris; Hoffding; Radhakrishnan; Russel; Alban G. Widgery, "Classical German Idealism: The Philosophy of Schopenhauer and Neo-Kantianism," in *A History of Philosophical Systems,* ed. V. Ferm (New York: The Philosophical Library, 1950).

7. Resources used in relation to post-Darwinian philosophy were Henri Bergson, *Creative Evolution,* trans. A. Mitchell (1907; rpt. New York: Random House, 1944); A. C. Bhattacharya, *Sri Aurobindo and Bergson* (Varanasi, India; Jagabhandu Prakashan, 1972); James K. Birx, *Pierre Teilhard de Chardin's Philosophy of Evolution* (Springfield, MA: Charles C. Thomas, 1972); Bonifazi; Fuller; Harris; Hoffding; Radhakrishnan; Russell; Alfred North Whitehead, *Process and Reality* (New York: Macmillan, 1927); C. F. Delaney, *Mind and Nature: A Study of the Naturalistic Philosophy of Cohen, Woodbridge and Sellars* (Notre Dame: University of Notre Dame Press, 1969).

THE MATERIALIST VIEW OF EVOLUTION

MONOD'S OVERALL VIEW

Jacques Monod, winner of the 1965 Nobel Prize for medicine and physiology, expounds his natural philosophy in the book *Chance and Necessity*.[1] Monod bases his view of biological evolution on the "postulate of objectivity," an a priori assumption that nature is utterly devoid of purpose. This postulate systematically denies that " 'true' knowledge can be got at by interpreting phenomena in terms of final causes—that is to say, of 'purpose' " (Monod, p. 21). Monod claims that since Galileo and Newton, science has always held this assumption and that because it has achieved such success in the technological realm by functioning according to this principle, "there is no way to be rid of it, even tentatively or in a limited area, without departing from the domain of science itself" (Monod, p. 21).

When one objectively observes living organisms, however, their goal-directedness is undeniable. Monod's effort is to account for this apparent purposiveness of living organisms and their evolution in objectively mechanistic terms. The "teleonomic character" of organisms resides in their ability to pursue the goal of preservation of the species, by reproducing their structural norm contained in DNA. Evolution, then, is a process of steady refinement in the teleonomic structure of living organisms. It is not a purposive process, for it is based on random mutations in DNA, which are judged by natural selection.

Monod discusses the difference between life and nonlife rather extensively, and his conclusion on the matter is a quantitative, rather than a qualitative, distinction. Living organisms are initially characterized as having two unique characteristics, teleonomy and reproductive invariance. However, teleonomy presents a "profound epistemological contradiction" to the postulate of objectivity. Monod devotes an entire chapter, therefore, to justifying "the single hypothesis that modern science here deems acceptable; namely, that invariance necessarily precedes teleonomy" (Monod, p. 23). Thus, he tries to eliminate teleonomy as an essential characteristic of living beings. He has already shown that certain nonliving entities, such as crystals, possess the property of reproductive invariance; ultimately, he arrives at the claim that the only difference between life and nonlife is in the quantity of information that must be invariantly reproduced.

Monod favors the theory of natural selection because it "is the only one so far proposed that is consistent with the postulate of objectivity" (Monod, p. 24). Natural selection judges the effects of chance genetic mutations according to their reproductive success—that is, according to how they affect the teleonomic performance of the organism. Mutations are random; that is, they are "fortuitous, and utterly without relation to whatever may be their effects upon teleonomic functioning" (Monod, p. 118). But whether or not a mutation is integrated into the organismic system depends upon its compatibility with the whole of the system already controlled by its teleonomic purpose. Selection judges teleonomic performance; this is why evolution appears to be purposive. The role of teleonomy in evolution will be discussed further in the section describing Monod's teleological position.

Some philosophers have made much of the point that biological evolution seems to contradict the second law of thermodynamics. This basic principle of physics states that for irreversible processes there is an increase in entropy—energy is being lost in the form of heat and, therefore, is always becoming less available. One implication of the second law is that the universe is becoming more disordered and homogenous, for it requires energy to maintain order and complexity. Monod explains the apparent contradictions to the second law presented by life's order-maintaining properties in three different ways. First, he points out that the temporal irreversibility of biological evolution is an expression of the second law. He also maintains, however, that purely by chance, life has managed to reascend the slope of entropy, temporarily stepping backward in time by means of natural selection. Monod takes still another approach to the energetics of life and evolution in his description of enzymatics. He claims that life's creation of order is the result of its proteins' ability to form stereospecific, noncovalent complexes, which are compatible with the second law.

Monod's philosophical intent in all three explanations of the energetics

of evolution is to show that there are no invisible forces or purposes direc-
ting the evolutionary process, that it can be explained by objective, entropic
chemical mechanisms. Indeed, for Monod, evolution is not a primary
characteristic of life, because it is generated by random imperfections in a
fundamentally invariant realm.

MONOD'S ONTOLOGY

The primacy of reproducive invariance over teleonomy is the central tenet
of Monod's ontology. It is, as has been shown, a necessary result of the a
priori assumption of the objectivity of nature, because the DNA replication
and translation system has been explained in completely mechanistic terms.
Monod has not reduced teleonomy to a completely physical or chemical explanation, but he firmly believes that "the ultimate interpretation of the most
distinctive properties of living beings" rests on the ability of proteins to form
stereospecific, noncovalent complexes (Monod, p. 61). Despite the belief,
Monod still insists that invariance precedes teleonomy, and devotes a chapter
to the functioning of DNA, which is called the fundamental biological invariant, DNA forms an "intensely conservative" system, "locked into itself,
utterly impervious ot any 'hints' from the outside world" (Monod, p. 110).
There is a one-way, completely deterministic relationship between DNA and
proteins (which are the agents of teleonomy). The DNA decoding mechanism
determines the amino acid sequence of the protein molecules, which in turn
determines their functioning. This is one sense, then, in which invariance
precedes teleonomy.

Monod characterizes the invariance of DNA as the Platonic element of
science. Stable species and mechanistic chemical pathways reveal universal
forms that make the diversity of life a paradox. In fact, evolution itself is
the result of fortuitous errors in an essentially changeless basic unit, the DNA
molecule.

Living organisms, then, are chemical machines, albeit self-constructing
machines, which are autonomously governed by internal chemical regulatory
processes:

> Hence they are proteins which channel the activity of the chemical machine, assure
> its coherent functioning, and put it together. All these teleonomic performances
> rest...upon the proteins'...ability to "recognize" other molecules...by their
> shape...At work here is, quite literally, a microscopic discriminative (if not
> "cognitive") faculty. (Monod, p. 46)

One ontological problem created by the primacy of invariance is the
undeniable phenomenon of change and evolution in nature. Monod's answer
to the ontological question "What is it that evolves?" would be not DNA,

or proteins, but the teleonomic functioning of organisms. The mutations that occur in the DNA molecule are completely random, but it is the teleonomic apparatus that "in evolution has acted as both guide and brake, and has retained, amplified, and integrated only a tiny fraction of the myriad opportunities offered it by nature's roulette" (Monod, p. 122). Every novelty is tested for its compatibility with the organism's projective purpose.

Here Monod has brought the reader face-to-face with a contradiction that must be resolved before the primacy of invariance can be affirmed. Monod states early in his book that the selective theory of evolution ranks "teleonomy as a secondary property deriving from invariance," hence assuring the objectivity of nature. However, in the chapter on evolution, the role of the teleonomic filter is given prime importance in providing the initial screening of genetic mutations. In addition, it is teleonomic performance itself that is judged by selection. Monod, then, appears ultimately to be confirming what he calls the vitalist and animist hypothesis: "*invariance is safeguarded, ontogeny guided,* and *evolution oriented* by an initial teleonomic principle" (Monod, p. 24).

Monod''s attempt to resolve this contradiction, at one point, focuses on the conflict in biological theory between reductionism and holism. His interpretation of holism is that it is opposed to any analysis of a system's parts. He presents three arguments in favor of chemical analysis. First, single protein molecules, not only complex systems, are capable of teleonomic performance. Second, the concept of gratuity explains the selective choice of molecular regulatory interactions according to their contribution to the coherence of the system. Third, microscopic cybernetic analysis shows that "all the activities that contribute to the growth and multiplication of that cell are interconnected and intercontrolled, directly or otherwise" (Monod, p. 80).

Monod carries the chemical reduction of organismic development as far as current research has progressed. He admits that many phenomena of life have yet to be explained in chemical terms; among these are morphogenesis (embryonic development), the origin of life, the inner workings of the human central nervous system, and various long-distance interactions within and among organisms. Monod expresses complete faith that all these phenomena will ultimately be accounted for by the properties and interactions of proteins, which themselves are the result of random chemical events preserved in the invariant DNA system.

Thus far, Monod's ontology has been discussed in regard to nonhuman organisms, and it has been shown that the postulate of objectivity requires that all their properties be explained mechanistically be reducing them to randomly originating chemical processes. When the focus of attention turns to the human being, however, a radical change in outlook occurs, which can be characterized as a dualist Cartesian metaphysic. The human brain is characterized by the unique development of the simulative function—the imagination of external events and programs of action. Symbolic language translates the subjective simulations of an individual so that they can be communicated to others; it is totally unlike animal communication. Monod admits that these higher cortical functions elude mechanical analysis, and he allows the possibility that the human mind is a qualitatively new phenomenon:

> Objective analysis obliges us to see that this seeming duality between body and mind within us is an illusion. But it is so well within, so intimately rooted in our being, that nothing could be vainer than to hope to dissipate it in the immediate awareness of subjectivity, or to learn to live emotionally or morally without it. And, besides, why should one have to? What doubt can there be of the presence of the spirit within us? (Monod, p. 159)

In summary, Monod's ontology of evolution proposes that it is teleonomic structures that are evolving. Despite their apparently purposive and holistic behavior, organisms can ultimately be explained as chemical machines whose functioning can be analyzed by examining interactions among cellular proteins, and whose development is based on blind, random mutations in the primary invariant, DNA. There is a quantitative difference only between life and nonlife, and between life and the human mind a qualitative change may have occurred, because human subjective awareness appears to defy chemical analysis. The postulate of objectivity requires that no purpose be attributed to natural processes. The "cognitive" qualities of proteins are due to their ability to recognize other molecules by their shape alone. Monod's ontology can best be described as a synthesis of early Greek atomism and Cartesian dualism, the result being a 20th-century materialistic view of the evolving units of the world.

MONOD'S TELEOLOGY

Despite his use of the term "teleonomic," Monod must reject any teleological view of nature and its evolution. The postulate of objectivity, a priori, demands this; but Monod also wants to support this rejection of teleology by emphasizing the basic operation of chance in living, evolving processes. Chance is the law governing the assembly of the amino acid sequence of proteins. The amino acid sequence is random in the sense that it is impossible to form a rule that could predict the next amino acid on any polypeptide chain, even if all the preceding ones are known. "Randomness caught on the wing, preserved, reproduced by the machinery of invariance and thus converted into order, rule, necessity. . . In the ontogenesis of a functional protein are reflected the origin and descent of the whole biosphere" (Monod, p. 98).

Chance is also at the root of evolution, because the mutations in DNA, the repository of the organism's heredity, are random occurrences. By "chance" mutations, Monod means that there is complete independence "between the occurrences that can provoke or permit an error in the replication of the genetic message and its functional consequences..." (Monod, p. 114). However, as was explained in the previous section, it is the teleonomic apparatus—how its function is affected by the mutation—that initially admits or rejects the innovation. The final judge of the mutation is selection, using the criterion of reproductive success.

Monod does not interpret natural selection as being related only to the conditions of the external environment. The interaction between an organism and its environment helps to determine the nature of the selective pressure it experiences. "Choices" of a certain behavior by an organism or species are often decisive factors in orienting selective pressures toward a continuous suuport of this behavior. For example, because a primitive fish "chose" to explore on land, selective pressures eventually engendered the powerful quadruped extremities, "fulfilling, extending, and amplifying the ancestral fish's hankering, its dream" (Monod, p. 127).

It is this relationship between an organism's behavior and natural selection that provides the key to what Monod calls the second evolution, in the human species, in which a teleological prospect becomes possible. This teleological prospect lies in the evolution of ideas, which will now be discussed as a central tenet of Monod's teleology.

The most rudimentary symbolic communication executed by one individual among the ancestors of modern man was a crucial choice that gave rise to heavy selective pressures favoring the development of linguistic ability, the brain, and "a special kind of intelligence." This was because these three areas enormous selective advantage, which by Monod's own criterion must be their reproductive success. Linguistic and cognitive patterns gradually became encoded in the genes, imprinted by the cumulative experience of the species. Symbolic language, in turn, opened the door for ideational and cultural evolution.

Although a totally blind process based on purely random events has produced man, his self-awareness and capacity to understand this truth make it possible for him to shape his own future evolution. Here again can be seen a striking shift in viewpoint, which is strongly suggestive of the Cartesian body/mind, man/nature dualism. Ideas, systems of thought, and culture form the evolution over which man now can gain control.

For a long time, ideational evolution kept only a step ahead of physical evolution; but gradually the central nervous system released its restraints, and ideational evolution became increasingly dependent and dominant. The human need to find meaning in existence was favored by natural selection and became genetic, because the experience of meaningfulness and purposiveness validated and anchored the social structure. This is why religions and philosophical systems have kept a tenacious hold on human culture. There is no truth in these ideational forms of meaning—only biological usefulness.

However, Monod maintains that the only ideational form capable of guiding the modern world's evolution is scientific, objective knowledge. Objective knowledge denies any meaning or purpose to human life; it teaches that man must "wake to his total solitude, his fundamental isolation. Now does he at last realize that, like a gypsy, he lives on the boundary of an alien world" (Monod, pp. 172–73). The crucial choice of scientific practice, because of its enormous material benefits, requires that ideational evolution be redirected so that objectivity is accepted not only as a methodological premise, but also as an epistemological and metaphysical premise.

Objective knowledge is excused from Monod's denial of truth to human ideas. Although it is itself an arbitrary metaphysical choice, the principle of objectivity is held to be the only "authentic" source of truth. Its authenticity lies in acknowledging and preserving the distinction between values and knowledge. It is revealing in this regard when Monod states that Descartes's *Discourse on Method* must be read as a moral meditation, for it is in the separation of knowledge and values that Cartesian dualism finds one of its most persistent manifestations. However, Monod appears to mix these categories by espousing an "ethic of knowledge," which holds his "true knowledge" to be a "transcendent value":

> It is obvious that the positing of the principle of objectivity as the condition of true knowledge *constitutes an ethical choice and not a judgment arrived at from knowledge since, according to the postulate's own terms, there cannot have been any 'true' knowledge prior to this arbitral choice.* In order to establish the *norm* for knowledge the objectivity principle defines a *value;* that value is objective knowledge itself. Thus, assenting to the principle of objectivity one announces one's adherence to the basic statement of an ethical system, one asserts *the ethic of knowledge.* (Monod, p. 176)

The ethic of knowledge will be dedicated to the kingdom of objectivity, which will allow man to live authentically. Inauthentic religious and philosophical systems have interfered with the work of natural selection, having allowed the genetic degradation of the human species. "Conditions of nonselection (or of selection-in-reverse) like those reigning in the advanced societies are a definite peril to the species" (Monod, p. 164). However, Monod belies that mankind's spiritual affliction is more dangerous than its genetic degradation. This malady of the spirit is caused by the attempt to cling to the old values of the animist tradition, while enjoying the material benefits of objective knowledge, which itself subverts the traditional values. The remedy is for humanity to embrace the ethic of knowledge, which will further enhance the evolution of "the transcendent kingdom of ideas, of knowledge, and of creation" (Monod, p. 180).

CRITICAL ANALYSIS OF MONOD'S OVERALL VIEW

A critical analysis of Monod's evolutionary metaphysic may appropriately begin with his primary a priori assumption, the postulate of objectivity. It is undeniable that this postulate has traditionally been adopted by scientists as a methodological assumption. Eliminating final causation, purposiveness, or invisible forces in the phenomena under investigation has been considered necessary for experimental methods designed according to mechanistic, quantitative rules. This methodological objectivity has been most successful in the physical sciences; in the biological and human sciences, it has achieved only limited success. This is why there exists the debate between holists and reductionists Monod refers to, and why it is essential that he assign a secondary role to teleonomy and attempt to reduce it to the chemical activity of proteins. It is his insecurity about the adequacy of his reduction of teleonomy that impels him to insist on the primacy of invariance. This insecurity is well founded, for the overall impact of Monod's book is the understanding that proteins themselves, as well as teleonomic systems, are endowed with qualities of cognition and purposiveness that play the major role in preservation of the species and evolution.

Monod calls upon the postulate of objectivity to defend the primacy of invariance over teleonomy, which he then uses to support the postulate of objectivity. Thus, Monod commits the logical fallacy of a petitio principii, in which a premise which is to be proved is implicitly taken for granted.[2] Despite his efforts to eliminate the purposive nature of living organisms, Monod must ultimately call upon his own faith in the future ability of molecular biologists to complete the task. He admits that many areas of organismic functioning still defy mechanistic analysis. This is why the postulate of objectivity must be made an a priori assumption.

As explained earlier, Monod's depiction of the relationship between evolution and entropy vacillates between maintaining that life and evolution are entropic processes and viewing them as temporary breaches of the second law of thermodynamics. Bertalanffy and Weiss present widely accepted arguments supporting the view of life and evolution as negentropic processes.[3] The thermodynamics of living systems is exceedingly complex and is just beginning to receive clarification by physicists such as Prigogine.[4] Nature is now viewed as an open system, whereas the second law is valid for closed systems only. Open systems are inherently negentropic. The philosophical problem involved in Monod's view is how order (negentropy) is produced by random events, without resort to purposiveness or to holistic phenomena, which operate on the system level rather than at the molecular level. Monod himself must resort to these concepts.

Another related philosophic problem in Monod's view of the thermodynamics of life is the origin of a self-replicating molecule. The initial formation of a DNA prototype would have the second law. Bertalanffy (1969) postulates that this must have required the presence of organizing forces or, in other words, a teleonomic system. Monod cites experiments demonstrating that the structural elements of DNA can form spontaneously in vitro. However, the separate elements were parts of a DNA molecule before they were broken up, so the presence of an underlying teleonomic tendency cannot be dismissed. In the words of biologist Paul Weiss, "You cheat by not mentioning the fact that you borrowed something from another system which was not the kind of system you are trying to explain." (Weiss, p. 45). Monod acknowledges that the chances were virtually zero that a random association of elements would form a prototypical nucleic acid. Most biologists and philosophers have turned to other explanations of the origin of life.[5]

It is remarkable that materialistic philosophers so firmly deny the existence of holistic or organizing forces in favor of zero-probability explanations. Many other "invisible" forces, such as electromagnetism and gravity, have been accepted. The difficulty appears to be in measurement, which is largely a problem of instrumentation. David Bohm, professor of theoretical physics at Birkbeck College, London, discusses how the use of lenses biased modern scientific theories toward analytic, rather than synthetic, approaches.[6] Lenses operate by separating into and focusing on the parts of the entity. This bias toward analysis has undoubtedly influenced the materialists' refusal to consider forces that may be holistic in nature. Monod implies that holistic schools of thought deny the value of the analytic approach to complex living systems. This is not the view of most holistic philosophers; what is usually claimed is that the whole displays properties qualitatively different from a simple summation of its parts.[7]

CRITICAL ANALYSIS OF MONOD'S ONTOLOGY

As indicated earlier, Monod's ontological position rests on his view of the relationship between invariance and teleonomy. The fallacy of the petitio principii has already been pointed out in connection with his choice of the primacy of invariance. Dewey discusses such a search for invariant entities in nature as a "bias in favor of objects of contemplative enjoyment, together with a theory that such objects are the adequate subject matter of science."[8] Biological philosopher U. J. Jensen refers to this same tendency, specifically among geneticists, to reify certain abstract terms (such as "genes"), and then to utilize the abstraction as an "ideal of indivisible particulateness."[9] This is precisely the problem with Monod's ontology. Reductionism and objectivity are elevated from their appropriate role as methodological tenets into ultimate metaphysical principles.

Monod's heavy emphasis on the invariant properties of DNA and their major function in life processes is, in itself, not completely accurate. "Contemporary geneticists believe that species stability is something of a myth; that the DNA of a species continually changes in small ways from one generation to another."[10] It is also now felt that external environmental influences control the expression of individual genes and sets of genes. DNA replication itself requires the influence of enzymes.[11] In addition, Monod points out that the functional equivalent of mechanical genetic transmission occurs in such nonliving entities as crystals; therefore, invariant reproduction cannot properly be used as the primary characteristic of life. Monod himself acknowledges the secondary role played by the DNA replication system in evolution; this role was discussed earlier in the chapter, in connection with the major role played by the teleonomic filter in natural selection. Ultimately, Monod must call on faith to support his view that the complex teleonomy of living organism can be accounted for solely by invariant genetic mechanisms.

To understand the inadequacy of explaining living organisms in terms of the genetic code, compare the DNA molecule to a string of words (as Monod, himself, does). The words can be translated mechanically from one language to another (into the language of the amino acid sequences), but there is higher-level dimension of grammar and syntax embedded in the words, and this dimension conveys its information only when the sentence or paragraph as a whole is apprehended. This dimension is analogous to organismic teleonomy, and Monod relegates it to a secondary status. But without it, one is faced with a meaningless string of molecules, as if one had a book but no mind to read and comprehend it.

Monod's rejection of a qualitative difference in favor of merely a quantitative difference between life and nonlife is a characteristic materialistic metaphysic. Quantification is the basis of materialistic analysis. Descartes's distinction between primary and secondary qualities, and the exclusion of the latter from the realm of science, has led to this bias. The primary qualities are those that can be mathematically defined and are felt to constitute the essential reality of an entity. Secondary qualities, perceptible by the senses (such as color, sound, smell, and the like), are regarded as being dependent on the mind of the perceiver.[12]

The doctrine of primary and secondary qualities is a direct consequence of conceiving nature to be mechanical. For Descartes, created reality consists of two substances, that which is extended (matter) and that which thins (mind). Consciousness is totally confined to the human mind, being excluded completely from matter. This is precisely what Monod is asserting in the postulate of objectivity, which he does not apply to the subjective experience of human beings

Thus, Monod is able to speak of living organisms as chemical machines. However, the very concept of development is fatal to this reductive materialism. Machines cannot evolve by themselves, cannot choose to become something different or to try a new behavior. Monod's depiction of the primitive fish choosing to explore the terra firma and his entire discussion of teleonomy and evolution carry him far beyond his materialistic presuppositions. Try as he will, he is unable to eliminate the attribution of cognition purposiveness even to the building blocks of life, the proteins. He is guilty of his own charge of animist projection.

The ontological dualism between mind and matter implicitly accepted by Monod has presented serious epistemological difficulties ever since Descartes explicated the position. Lewis provides a clear depiction of Monod's Cartesian stance:

> Monod never attempts to justify his belief in the spiritual world on rational grounds. He appeals only to existential choice as its basis, and to arbitrary ethical postulates as the basis of morals and social life. This is hardly different from Descartes' "clearn and distinct ideas"... Their basis is only what this man or that man *feels* to be indubitable.[13]

At various points in his treatise, Monod resorts to three classical solutions to the epistemological problem of Cartesian dualism, the relation between the mind and the body. His discussion of the influence exerted by man's linguistic and cognitive capacity on the physical evolution of the brain appears to be interactionism. His final extolment of the reality of subjective consciousness suggests parallelism. And, finally, his faith that all the phenomena of life and mind can be attributed to the chemical properties of proteins developed by blind chance results in epiphenomenalism. Insofar as Monod proves this last case, he has invalidated his conclusions entirely, for then he cannot exempt any theory, even the postulate of objectivity, from its basis in random, meaningless errors in the genetic code. There remain no grounds for suposing that his arguments are correct (Lewis, pp. 33–35).

Monod's ontological problems are further compounded by his support of a Kantian epistemology at a certain point in his book. It appears that he is trying to reconcile a Cartesian and Kantian view of the innateness of ideas with the empiricist position that all ideas are derived from sensations of the external world. His reconciliation can be summarized as follows: our cognitive patterns or forms are genetically innate, having evolved from the cumulative experience of the species in its dealings with the environment; hence, they provide the individual with "a representation of the material world adequate for the performance of the species" (Monod, p. 154). The epistemological aspects of this view will be discussed in the critique of Monod's teleological position. At this point, the ontological implications require closer examination.

The essential ontological difficulty of body/mind dualism is left unresolved by Monod's view; in fact, it is brought into glaring relief. How can the DNA molecule, via the cellular proteins, create or influence cognitive processes? As long as the postulate of objectivity remains in effect, what is necessarily implied is a purely physical entity producing a mental condition. And, conversely, how can cognitive experience become encoded in a physical molecule? One must conclude that in order to interact, these two aspects of nature must share certain characteristics. Or, as many philosophers have posited, they must be two aspects of a single underlying reality.

CRITICAL ANALYSIS OF MONOD'S TELEOLOGY

Monod's natural philosophy proposes two teleological views for two evolutions that are delineated—one for the nonhuman realm, and the other for the human realm. In the former arena of evolution, Monod holds, random mutation and natural selection provide a complete explanation of a process that is of only secondary importance in the fundamentally invariant world of nature. Chance (mutation) and necessity (selection), he feels, provide a completely mechanistic, nonteleological explanation of nonhuman evolution. However, many philosophers, as well as biologists, feel that the directionality of evolution is not adequately accounted for by these two factors alone.

One difficulty in attributing the extreme complexity of the higher animals to random processes is that the amount of time required to produce these creatures in this manner would be virtually infinite. Evolution appears to be a very slow process, but not when the magnitude of the changes and developments involved are considered. Seemingly insoluble problems are created by assuming that matter is a totally inert, passive substance. For this reason, many philosophers have suggested that the view of matter itself be modified to include an inner potential for transformation.[14]

Although Monod maintains that natural selection is the only evolutionary principle compatible with the postulate of objectivity, when he actually explains the contemporary refinement of the idea of selection, he attributes the major role in the selective process to the teleonomic apparatus. Still, the theory of natural selection presents several problems that require mention. Contemporary biologists have pointed out that many structures and behaviors that emerge in a species have little, if any, apparent selective advantage.[15] Indeed, many such features are so specialized and elaborate that they seem even to jeopardize the organism's survival value. The theory of natural selection exhibits the more serious logical flaw of tautology and circularity. It is tautologous, or self-defining, in that a selectionist explanation is always a posteriori (Bertalanffy, 1969). After an adaptational change occurs, it is explained as being a result of natural selection. The circularity of the theory lies in the fact that the selective process requires the characteristics of a living system, an integrated organism. Harris presents this point most clearly:

> Evolution by natural selection presumes variations in the progeny from some parental stock and the selection of the variants which are better adapted to environmental conditions...The prerequisite for natural selection, therefore, is an already existing whole, not less than a self-replicating protein molecule, which itself requires for its genesis a complex cycle of chemical reactions...and this is found to presuppose an already existing organization of living matter. Ordered totality is thus logically prior to natural selection.[16]

Thus, the problem of the origin of life remains unsolved, and the continuity of nature threatened.

A final emphasis of a critical point regarding the selective process must be made once again. If, indeed, it is the teleonomic system that has acted as the initial screener as well as the "guide and brake" in evolution, and the teleonomic system is goal-oriented, one is forced to view the directionality of evolution as a purposive, or teleological process.[17] By Monod's delineation of the teleonomic goal as one of species preservation, evolution has certainly failed in reaching its goal. Many biologists and philosophers, however, view the essential teleonomic goal of living systems as self-transcendence.[18] Others have clearly outlined the progressive development of consciousness as constituting the directionality of evolution from bacterium to man.[19]

In the realm of human evolution, Monod does allow for an evolution of consciousness or, in his terms, an evolution of ideas. Monod wants to account for ideational evolution also in terms of adaptation and natural selection. The burden falls upon him, then, to explain how the history of human ideas has supported the selective goal of reproductive invariance. Systems of thought, it is claimed, that provide a sense of meaning and purpose to life succeeded because they facilitated social cohesiveness and maintenance of the social order. How, then, does he justify their sudden abandonment?

Given this description of the biological usefulness of the traditional systems of thought, Monod's later attack of them as a threat to the species presents a paradox. Monod focuses on their altruistic tendencies, which soften the impact of natural selection. It is also the case that many ideologies have been devoted to reforming or overthrowing an established social order. Millions of human lives have been destroyed over ideational systems; this hardly seems to have served the purpose of preserving reproductive invariance. Also, the current trend of genetic and cultural mixing is hastening, rather than slowing down, the transformation of the species.

Monod provides no justification for the evolutionary value of "true knowledge" (objective knowledge), which he claims is the only ideational system capable of guiding mankind's further evolution. The only criterion he has provided for "evolutionary value" is the contribution to the invariant reproduction and preservation of the human species. The ethic of knowledge posits a meaningless, alien existence for humanity in the universe, and would appear to provide very little impetus for mankind to continue its purposeless existence. Objective knowledge is creating an existential crisis in modern man, and the only cure is to accept it arbitrarily, to elevate it to the status of religion by a leap of faith, and to pursue its ideal—objective knowledge itself. This hardly appears to be a convincing argument in support of a new metaphysical stance.

As was mentioned above, Monod gives no explanation of how the ethic of knowledge will contribute to the invariant preservation of the species. In fact, the development of objective knowledge without the constraints of a value system has placed mankind on the brink of self-destruction. If the objective knowledge developed to serve the purpose of natural selection, one can only conclude that selection has been a failure, its purpose having been defeated by its own products.

Monod realizes that no justification can be found for the ethic of knowledge other than its material benefits for certain segments of humanity, so he must attribute to his suggested teleological goal the qualities of a new religion. The language he uses to describe this new ethic echoes biblical phraseology— the kingdom of ideas, the new convenant, transcending the self, self-sacrifice. How this can be a valid reason for accepting the new religion over the old religions and philosophies rests upon an extremely ambiguous criterion of authenticity. Authenticity, for Monod, lies in the acknowledgment of the separation between knowledge and values, yet Monod's delineation of true knowledge is a value judgment as "inauthentic" as any of the animist philosophies.

Furthermore, the separation of knowledge and values is largely considered undesirable by modern philosophers. This dichotomy is based, ultimately, on the Cartesian split between mind and matter. Mending this split has been a priority for many contemporary philosophhers, following the lead of the earlier holistic approaches of Dewey and Whitehead.[20] Closely related to the issue of the dichotomy between knowledge and values is that between mechanism and teleology. Monod perceives any teleological explanation of evolution as a threat to the postulate of objectivity. Indeed, this is precisely what the postulate involves—the denial of teleology or purposiveness in natural processes. The issue of teleology versus mechanism has been debated since the Aristotelian doctrine of causation was developed. It may help to clarify it by turning to the insight of Russell.

Russell, himself one of the founders of modern materialism, maintains that teleological and mechanistic causation are not mutually exclusive, as Monod considers them to be:

> Now the fact—if it be a fact—that the universe is mechanical has no bearing on the question whether it is teleological...The question whether, or how far, our actual world is teleological, cannot, therefore, be settled by proving that it is mechanical, and the desire that it should be teleological is no ground for wishing it to be not mechanical...
>
> It may well be that the same system which is susceptible of material determinants is also susceptible of mental determinants; thus a mechanical system may be deter-mined by sets of volitions, as well as by sets of material facts.[21] Monod, however, apparently believes that the two aspects of causation are irreconcilable.

CONCLUSION

Monod's primary metaphysical tenet, the postulate of objectivity, is characteristic of the modern materialistic school of philosophy. Materialism was defined in chapter 1 as a philosophy holding all reality to be of the nature of matter. Monod's view of matter is that it is completely devoid of any purposiveness, or, ontologically, that it is devoid of mind. Monod is not, however, willing to deny the unique properties of mind in the human sphere of experience, although he does suggest that ultimately they will prove to be explainable in completely physicochemical terms. Thus, the reader is led into all the problems connected with a classical Cartesian dualism.

Harris has pointed out that the concept of evolution, in which an underlying continuity is established among all the stages of development in nature, requires a philosophy that can explain the emergence of mind without describing a discontinuity such as the one Monod resorts to.[22] Huxley, one of the leading proponents of the Neo-Darwinian view, poses the problem as being ''how we can come to terms scientifically with a reality which combines both material and mental properties in its unitary pattern.''[23] Monod provides no coherent solution to this ontological problem. He has taken a respected and effective methodological dictum of science and transplanted it into the realm of metaphysics, seemingly oblivious to the fact that science deals with only a limited, abstracted segment of reality. He has also taken one particular branch of science, biochemistry, and attempted to explain all the phenomena of nature, including evolution, in terms of its area of concern—cellular molecules. But Monod has been unable to account for the goal-oriented behavior of living organisms and their functioning as coherent, integrated wholes—much less the phenomenon of human consciousness—in purely biochemical terms. In his very language, Monod is unable to separate mind from matter, thus are found repeated references to the cognitive qualities of proteins.

Monod is on even weaker logical ground when he claims that the ethic of knowledge, which denies any ultimate purpose or meaning to human existence, must be accepted on purely arbitrary grounds because it is consistent with science's methodological postulate. He gives no reason for why or how this ethic will allow mankind to guide its further evolutionary course. If one accepts the materialist's reduction of cognition to fortuitous chemical processes, no truth can be claimed for any particular ideology. However, if one accepts the Cartesian split between mind and matter, the continuity of evolution is invalidated and there is no justification for applying descriptions of the material world to the world of human consciousness. These are the only two possibilities Monod's materialistic ontological and teleological views allow. We will now turn to an idealist alternative to the metaphysics of evolution, as expressed in the philosophy of Pierre Teilhard de Chardin.

REFERENCES

1. Jacques Monod, *Chance and Necessity,* trans. A. Wainhouse (New York; Knopf, 1971). All further references to this work appear in the text.

2. Guy Quintelier, ''Ideal Objectivity, Modern Biology and Technical

Innovation," *Man and World,* 14 (1981), 369–85.

3. Ludwig van Bertalanffy, "Chance or Law," and Paul Weiss, "The Living System," in *Beyond Reductionism,* ed. Arthur Koestler and J. R. Smythies (New York: Macmillan, 1969).

4. Ilya Prigogine, *From Being to Becoming* (San Francisco: Freeman, 1980).

5. Robert Shapiro, "The Origin of Life," manuscript submitted for publication, 1983.

6. David Bohm, *Wholeness and the Implicate Order* (London: Routledge & Kegan Paul, 1980), p. 144.

7. Ervin Laszlo, *The Systems View of the World* (New York: Braziller, 1972); P. Beurton, "Organismic Evolution and Subject-Object Dialectics," in *The Philosophy of Evolution,* ed. U. J. Jensen and R. Harre (New York: St. Martin's, 1981), pp. 45–60.

8. John Dewey, *Experience and Nature,* 2 ed. (1929; rpt. New York: Dover, 1958), p. 149.

9. U. J. Jensen, "Introduction: Preconditions for Evolutionary Thinking," in *The Philosophy of Evolution,* ed. U. J. Jensen, p. 14.

10. Robin E. Monro, "Interpreting Molecular Biology," in *Beyond Chance and Necessity,* ed. John Lewis (Atlantic Highlands, NJ: Humanities Press, 1974), p. 106.

11. C. H. Waddington, "How Much Is Evolution Affected by Chance and Necessity?" in *Beyond Chance and Necessity,* pp. 89–102.

12. René Descartes, *Meditations on First Philosophy,* III, trans. Elizabeth S. Haldane and G. R. T. Ross, from 2nd Latin ed. (1642), in *The Philosophical Works of Descartes* (1911; rpt. Cambridge: Cambridge University Press, 1972), Vol. I.

13. John Lewis, "The Cartesian Paradox," in *Beyond Chance and Necessity,* p. 38.

14. See, for example; Bergson, Jantsch, Leibniz, Melsen, and Whitehead; all in the Bibliography.

15. S. J. Gould and N. Eldredge, "Punctuated Equilibria: the Tempo and Mode of Evolution Reconsidered," *Paleobiology,* 3 (1977), 115–51.

16. Errol E. Harris, *The Foundations of Metaphysics in Science* (1965; rpt. Lanham, MD: University Press of America, 1983), pp. 194–96.

17. P. Beurton, "Organismic Evolution and Subject-Object Dialectics," in *The Philosophy of Evolution,* p. 56.

18. Erich Jantsch, "Unifying Principles of Evolution," in *The Evolutionary Vision,* ed. Erich Jantsch, AAAS Selected Symposia Series, 61 (Boulder, CO: Westview, 1981).

19. Theodosius Dobzhansky, "Two Contrasting World Views," in *Beyond Chance and Necessity;* Julian Huxley, *Evolution in Action* (1953; rpt. New York: Harper, 1966); Jantsch, "Unifying Principles;" Andrew van Melsen, *Evolution and Philosophy* (Pittsburgh: Dusquesne Univ. Press, 1965).

20. John Dewey, *Experience and Nature;* Alfred North Whitehead, *Process and Reality* (1929; rpt. New York: Harper, 1960).

21. Bertrand Russell, *Mysticism and Logic* (1917; rpt. New York: Double-day Anchor Books, n.d.), pp. 194–200.

22. Errol E. Harris, *Nature, Mind and Modern Science* (London: George Allen & Unwin, 1954).

23. Julian Huxley, *Evolution in Action,* p. 30.

4

THE IDEALIST VIEW OF EVOLUTION

TEILHARD'S OVERALL VIEW

For Pierre Teilhard de Chardin, evolution is a cosmic process, as well as a biological phenomenon. His focus is the primary flow of universal becoming, or cosmogenesis, and man's place in this flow. One of the most striking attributes of Teilhard's approach to evolution is the philosophical decision to assign paramount significance to human consciousness, which must be incorporated into the overall view of evolution. "We must make up our minds, by virtue of the general perspectives of evolution themselves, to make a special place in the physics of the universe for the powers of consciousness, spontaneity and improbability represented by life."[1]

Teilhard contends that materialistic attempts to account for the appearance of human consciousness by following evolution up from inert matter have failed. Therefore, he traces evolution back from man, and finds that even the most rudimentary elements of the universe must contain a "within" as well as a "without." Only in this way can the continuity and coherence of the universe be maintained; only then can the emergence of human mentality be explained.

Teilhard does not provide a consistent definition of the term "consciousness." He uses the terms "interiority," "immanence," and "spontaneity" to denote various qualities of consciousness. Perhaps the best meaning that can be ascribed to it, for Teilhard's purposes, is "awareness." Perception is the basis of awareness, existing in even the most basic interactions between elements and particles. Perception and interiority require and contribute to each other. Interiority implies awareness, which appears to be the consciousness of which Teilhard speaks.

The totality of human experience and the totality of the universe are included in Teilhard's view. Interiority, spontaneity, and freedom are the common experience of human beings, and cannot be dismissed from a complete desription of the world:

> If the cosmos were basically material, it would be physically incapable of containing man...Man's position in nature cannot be explained without a factor of psychic growth. No, the universe was not born without motion; its structure betrays (at least in the past) a global evolution of its mass towards an ever increasing interiorization.[2]

Teilhard describes evolution as an integrative process that manifests increasingly complex and centered forms, with each further degree of integration being accompanied by a growth of inner consciousness, spontaneity, and freedom. At the same time, Tielhard depicts all the evolutes in the universe as being coextensive with the totality, forming an essential unity that will be completely manifest at the end of the evolutionary process.

The critical axiom of Teilhard's view of evolution is the law of centro-complexity-consciousness. This law describes the direction of evolution as being toward increasing complexity, centration, interiority, and consciousness. Phenomenologically, Teilhard observes that consciousness appears to be an effect of complexity. Metaphysically, however, he holds the traditional idealist view that it is the urge of unfolding consciousness that impels the increasing complexity and centricity of the evolutes. Here is where Teilhard's view differs from those of Spencer and the critical naturalists, for they deny this primary role of consciousness.

Teilhard maintains that the law of centro-complexity-consciousness adds a new dimension to the traditional measurement domains of science. One standard dimension of scientific measurement ranges from the infinitesimal to the immense. The forces operating in the universe change radically as either of these extremes is approached. Common scientific measurement occurs within the middle range of this scale. Another traditional dimension of scientific measurement is that of speed. For example, Einstein's theory of relativity applies to objects whose speed approaches that of light. Teilhard insists that the dimension of complexity also be considered as one in which there is an intimate relationship between quantity and quality.

> A new cosmic milieu is created by the introduction of this additional dimension; and in this milieu the vitalization of matter immediately ceases to appear puzzling or inexplicable...Life is the property that is peculiar to *large organized*

numbers, it is the specific effect of matter carried to an extreme degree of internal structuration. (*AE,* pp. 29–30)

Human self-awareness, or reflexion, is another critical transition, or change of state, that occurs when complexity folds in completely on itself, becoming fully centered. The noosphere, the next stage of evolution, is currently forming by a synthesis of human minds into a single planetary organism, or "thinking envelope." This view of dimensional zones allows Teilhard to explain the evolutionary emergence of entirely new stages of development, while at the same time maintaining the underlying continuity of the process.

Teilhard discusses extensively the issue of entropy/negentropy in evolution. His view is essentially the opposite of Monod's, although in different writings slight variations can be noted. Phenomenologically, it appears that entropy and negentropy are two different currents in the universe, representing two different categories, such as matter and spirit. However, when Teilhard speaks metaphysically, he abandons phenomenological dualism in favor of an ontological monism, in which the synthesizing flow of negentropy is the significant cosmic event and entropy is at best a temporary eddy in the current. "Surely, if we really wish to unify the real, we should completely reverse the values— that is, we should consider the whole of thermodynamics as an untenable and ephemeral by-effect of the concentration on itself of what we call 'consciousness' " (*AE,* p. 393). Here one is reminded of Bergson's view that matter is a temporary back-flow in the current of the élan vital.

This view of negentropy is intimately related to Teilhard's view of the role played by chance in the evolutionary process. Chance undoubtedly plays the major part in the initial stages of evolution, but as matter becomes more complex, the process gradually becomes permeated by choice; it becomes elective rather than selective. Random events provide the necessary variety and diversity out of which the "energy of universal evolution" chooses arrangements that are increasingly ordered, complex, and centered. Explaining, as Monod does, all the phenomena of change and development in nature as the exclusive result of blind chance does not account for the identifiable trend toward increasing consciousness. Physical mutations are necessary, but not sufficient. "It is always only with the chances they make use of that [the cosmic organic centers] gradually build up the fabric of their finality...All life, and all thought, is simply the seizing and organizing of chance" (*AE,* pp. 136–7).

In summary, then, Teilhard sees the basic movement of evolution as being toward greater complexity, organization, centration, and consciousness. The diversity and differentiation of living forms provide the necessary opportunities allowing the evolutionary process to slowly advance into greater complexity and interiority. Having examined Teilhard's overall view of the evolutionary process, we present below the ontological and teleological aspects of his view.

TEILHARD'S ONTOLOGY

The primary assertion of Teilhard's ontology is that all energy—hence, all matter—is psychic in nature. The basic Weltstoff is characterized by immanence, a most rudimentary consciousness, which is mainly potentiality rather than actuality. The proof of this is that even at the subatomic level, particles or waves of energy react to and interact with each other. Reaction implies mutual perception; therefore, this interaction involves at least a minimum of interiority, or subjectivity.

Teilhard's "centrology" describes in detail the nature of his evolute in a style reminiscent of Leibniz's "monadology." Teilhard establishes a pluralistic monadism:

> At every degree of size and complexity, cosmic particles or grains are not simply, as physics has recognized, centers of universal dynamic radiation: all of them, in addition (rather like man), have and represent a small "within"...in which is reflected, at a more or less rudimentary stage, a particular representation of the world: in relation to themselves they are psychic centers—and at the same time they are infinitesimal psychic centers of the universe. In other words, consciousness is a universal molecular property; and the molecular state of the world is a manifestation of the pluralized state of some potentiality of universal consciousness. (*AE*, p. 101)

The centricity, or centeredness, of the elements of the universe provides the true measure of their consciousness. The universe is moved by a stream of centration, or integration; it has evolved from the fragmentary centricity of matter, through the closed-up centers of life, to the punctiform centricity of man. One can find a physical expression of this metaphysical schema in the fact that man and the "higher" forms of life are characterized by a central nervous system, whereas the lower forms have only a peripheral nervous system.

For Teilhard, centration occurs through union. In the realm of prelife, fragmentary centers (atoms) are gradually fused together (into molecules). In the domain of life, the embryonic organism unifies and centers the rapidly proliferating cells. In the human realm, the noosphere, the thinking envelope of the earth, is evolving from center-to-center contact among individuals, "by a direct tuning and resonance of their consciousness" (*AE*, p. 115). Therefore, the universal stream of becoming is a universal stream of union and centration.

Teilhard presents three "laws of union," which describe the properties of a world obeying the law of centro-complexity-consciousness. First, union creates. Second, union differentiates. Finally, union personalizes. Personalization is defined as creative differentiation, so the last law serves as a synthesis of the first two. The evolutionary trend toward complexity, centration, and unification finally becomes, then, a trend toward personalization, or creative differentiation. Underlying all of these qualities and processes is the basic Weltstoff, psychic energy, in its phases of elements, life, man, and society.

Human consciousness is distinctive in its quality of reflection, or self-awareness, which is the result of complete centration and personalization. Teilhard believes that the only evolute that survives death is the "human molecule," because of its capacity to enter into an ultimate personalizing union in Omega. Omega is the source and the goal of the evolving universe, an ultrapersonal, ultracentered Supreme Consciousness, which is immanent in, but also transcends, the various units of evolution. "In Omega, then, a maximum complexity, cosmic in extent, coincides with a maximum cosmic centricity" (*AE,* p. 111).

Although Teilhard occasionally refers, in a dualistic fashion, to matter and spirit, or tangential and radial energy, these seem to be phenomenological references rather than ontological categories. Tangential energy represents the forces of structural arrangement and chance variation that allow the proliferation of forms so important to the evolutionary process. Radial energy represents an inherent drive toward self-transcendence and more complex and centered forms, ensuring that the movement toward increasing consciousness is maintained. Evolutionary philosophers such as Morgan, Alexander, Bergson, and Whitehead have also postulated such a creative, immanent force in nature that underlies the advance toward higher forms. These two energies, tangential and radial, represent two modes of activity of the one energy composing the universe. At times Teilhard uses the term "spirit-matter" to describe the basic stuff of the universe, in an attempt to express the belief that these two modes of activity are inseparable, complementary, "no more than two aspects or phases of a single 'interiorizing arrangement'" (*AE,* pp. 258–59). In this study the term "conscious energy" is used to represent Teilhard's Weltstoff, for this term captures the philosopher's meaning without suggesting a metaphysical dualism.

Teilhard's ontology is the very antithesis of reductionism. Synthesis, rather than analysis, is his method. As mentioned earlier, the whole of human experience, from scientific to mystical, is included in this view:

> The whole phenomenon of consciousness, when submitted to scientific investigation, gives the impression of dissolving and melting away, like an illusion, in the uniform flood of a universal determinism...Surely, however, this is simply because their eyes are still closed to the fundamental and mutually opposed operation of synthesis and analysis in the general structure of the universe. (*AE,* p. 131)

Consciousness, or awareness, is a holistic phenomenon, and once it has been assigned to its proper place in the universe, Teilhard says, "it is radically impossible to conceive that 'interiorized' and spontaneous elements could ever have developed from a universe presumed in its initial state to have consisted entirely of determinisms" (*HE,* p. 23). A materialistic ontology cannot support a Teilhardian view of the evolution of consciousness.

TEILHARD'S TELEOLOGY

Teilhard's teleology is perhaps the most distinctive aspect of his evolutionary philosophy. The philosopher identifies several seemingly contradictory trends, which must be clarified in connection with his teleology. Union and individuality, involution and evolution, immanence and transcendence are synthesized to provide a picture of the evolutionary process that incorporates scientific observation as well as the philosopher's personal mystical experience. The following discussion will focus on the theme of personalization, which has been taken to be the central tenet of Teilhard's teleological outlook.

As has already been explained, Teilhard believes that it is conscious energy that is evolving in the universal becoming. The direction, or goal, of evolution is the concern of a teleological analysis. For man—who is at the leading edge of the evolutionary process, according to Teilhard—the direction is toward a universal or cosmic consciousness that is ultrapersonalizing rather than self-annihilating. This paradox is explained by the axiom presented above: union personalizes. Union is the mechanism by which evolution is occurring—union among mankind and, at the same time, union with an Ultimate Reality. At the human level, union is an evolution of consciousness beyond the stage of mind, into an awareness of the essential unity of the universe. The awareness to which Teilhard refers has been recognized by numerous philosphers, as was seen in the historical review for this study. It is felt to be a higher, more evolved, consciousness, which reveals aspects of reality that transcend the divisions of space and time. Teilhard believes that mankind as a whole, and an ever-increasing number of individuals, are developing this consciousness. Many Western idealists have seen reason as the highest possible mode of consciousness; for Teilhard, reason is to be transcended.

In Teilhard's teleological view, the evolution of consciousness is a cosmic process of personalization. Individuality, in the sense of separateness, decreases; but personality, in the sense of being profoundly oneself, increases. Differentiation is an effect of union. For example, the union of billions of cells in the human body is accompanied by an exceedingly elaborate differentiation of the cells into various tissues and organs. Therefore, according to Teilhard, full personalization will occur only when mankind converges, uniting into an organic whole:

> Other spheres must exist in the future and, inevitably, a supreme center in which all the personal energy represented by human consciousness must be gathered and 'super-personalized.' We are moving towards a higher state of general consciousness, which is linked with a futher synthesis of our particular consciousness. (*HE,* p. 103)

Teilhard provides evidence of the convergence, or union, of mankind from several modern phenomena. The collaborative effort of scientific research, which transcends national boundaries, is a powerful source of inspiration to him. He sees global communication networks, international business endeavors, cultural exchange and mixing, the United Nations, and even the World Wars as manifestations of "totalization," the development of a planetary human organism. Teilhard does not ignore or dismiss the recognition that totalization can become a stifling, depersonalizing experience. He makes it clear that a deep affective relationship of love must evolve along with "planetization." This love must be a universal affection among human beings. "By its nature, love is the only synthesizing energy whose differentiating action can super-personalize us" (*AE,* p. 47).

Teilhard asserts that human consciousness, because of its reflective (self-aware) nature, demands and receives immortality. If the universe were to deny man irreversibility of consciousness, it would be structurally absurd; if a self-aware species learns that it has no future beyond death, it will lose all motivation for participating in the evolutionary process. "It is physically impossible for the universe simultaneously to contain in itself both a reflective activity and a total death. . . Evolution, struck at its very heart by self-disgust, automatically comes to a halt in a meaningless universe" (*AE,* pp. 41–43).

Teilhard's conception of a universal consciousness, Omega, which is both the source and the end of the evolving cosmos, has been espoused by such philosophers as Plato, Plotinus, Spinoza, Hegel, Schelling, Bergson, and Whitehead. Generally, some sort of an involution of the Absolute or Eternal into the world of becoming is suggested in these metaphysical systems, followed by an evolution back into the Absolute. Teilhard does not support a classical Aristotelian final causation in his teleology, however; this would involve the view that evolution is being directed by the Absolute end or goal. Teilhard places the driving force of evolution within the evolutes, innate in the conscious energy of the cosmos. The creative impulse toward self-transcendence, into more complex and conscious entities, is immanent in the Weltstoff:

> Matter is affected in its entirety by metamorphosis. Moreover, just because this metamorphosis extends by right to the whole imaginable expanse of reality, no external cause seems experimentally assignable for the transformation's occurence. We are in the presence of a kind of autonomous process and inner spontaneity. (*HE,* p. 97)

Because man has the capacity to understand the evolutionary process, he also has the choice of promoting or hindering its progress. Freedom increases with evolving consciousness. Conscious participation is every individual's evolutionary heritage and responsibility.

CRITIQUE OF TEILHARD'S OVERALL VIEW

The major philosophical decision Teilhard makes is assigning consciousness a primary role in the universal schema. His arguments for this decision are

persuasive, revolving around his interpretation of the philosophical requirement of coherence:

> If the construction does not form a complete whole, or if it contradicts some part
> of experience, it will show that the initial hypothesis was bad and should be aban-
> doned. But if, on the contrary, it seems to encircle and harmonize the world to
> a greater degree, then we must conclude that...we have come near to the truth.
> The *truth* is nothing but the total coherence of the universe in relation to each
> part of itself. (*HE,* p. 54)

Teilhard's understanding of philosophical coherence is consistent with Price's
statement that "what is demanded of the speculative metaphysician is just
a unifying conception...What the metaphysician has to show is that his
method or arrangement—his principle of systematic representation—is a
possible one."[3]

Consciousess, or interiority, is indeed an undeniable and major aspect of
the human experience. Many philosophers have chosen to minimize its importance in the larger universe, however, drawing on comparisons between
the spatial and temporal minuteness of the human species against the vastness
of the cosmos. However, a consciousness that can extend infinitely in space
and time and can also transcend space and time, which can even partially
comprehend the vastness to which it is comparing itself, is qualitatively, if
not quantitatively, of enormous significance. To deny its importance appears
to be an avoidance of the problems involved in incorporating it into a comprehensive philosophical outlook. A coherent metaphysical system, then, must
be able to explain the phenomenon of consciousness.

Teilhard's explanation of the connection between complexity and consciousness via the mechanism of centration deserves attention because of its
heuristic value. This, it must be remembered, is a metaphysical rather than
a scientific explanation; but it finds support from the realm of biological
science. Increasingly complex forms of life are characterized by increasing
differentiation and centration. The central nervous system of the primates
and man is a clear example of this centration. Integration allows the unit
to function as a whole, to experience a "within" and a "without." The within
is what perceives and interacts with the without. Perception implies
consciousness; thus the logical-empirical connection between complexity and
consciousness appears solid.

Teilhard's emergentism is another acceptable aspect of his overall view
of evolution. By linking the emergence of new forms and stages of evolution
with increasing complexity and centricity, he allows creative novelty without
sacrificing the continuity of the material process. This approach is not unique
to Teilhard; in fact, it is characteristic of the modern naturalistic philosophy
espoused by Sellars, and of the earlier evolutionary philosophers Morgan,
Alexander, and Smuts. The concepts of evolutionary emergence allows for
the appearance of new qualitative properties, such as life and mind, in

connection with certain quantitative thresholds. Vitalistic theses, which postulate the entrance of outside forces into matter, can be avoided.

More recently, Prigogine's view of evolution as an example of dissipative self-organization in nonequilibrium systems has been elaborated by Jantsch to describe an evolutionary principle of "anagenisis." This refers to the evolution of evolutionary dynamics themselves, which brings into play qualitatively new levels of envolving systems.[4] When change in a living system or its environment reaches a critical threshold, the system is challenged to reach a new state of organization or to face dissolution. Evolution, then, is seen as a process of system self-organization through perturbation and creative response. This paradigm appears to support the earlier views of Teilhard and the above-mentioned philosophers who described evolutionary emergence. Teilhard's language anticipates Prigogine's:

> When matter has reached certain extreme levels of transformation, then an extremely small modification in its arrangements (or in the conditions that govern the arrangements) allows it suddenly to modify its properties or even to change its state. This [is the] notion of critical thresholds. (*AE*, p. 284)

Evolutionary emergence provides a more convincing explanation of the various orders of life than does Monod's reduction of all differences to cellular biochemical processes. It is a holistic approach that looks at the total system and its environment. To review, Monod's point of view is that there is no qualitative difference among the various orders of molecules, plants, animals, and man. The difference lies only in the quantity of information transmitted teleonomically. Dissatisfaction with this reductionistic explanation has led to the current interest in evolutionary processes involving self-transcendence, "the creative reaching out of a system beyond its own physical and mental bound."[5]

CRITIQUE OF TEILHARD'S ONTOLOGY

As described earlier, Teilhard's essential ontological thesis is that energy is consciousness. This seems at first glance to be a radical view that contradicts the traditional Cartesian description of matter as inert particles characterized only by extension. Its radicalness loses its intensity, however, when the current scientific views of matter and energy are examined. Cartesian materialism has long been dead in the community of scientists. Bernhard Rensch, director of the Institute of Zoology at the University of Muenster and a preeminent biophilosopher, has maintained that molecules, atoms, and elementary particles are protopsychical in character:

We now think quite differently about the "solidity" of the matter from which the living organism is made up. "Solid substance" has now given place to fields of energy, and these can only be comprehended in terms of relationships. This conception makes it easier to incorporate the findings of physics in a panpsychistic, identistic picture.[6]

For Rensch, the evolution of matter is also the evolution of consciousness.

Bohm similarly comments on the philosophical implications of the Cartesian view of matter:

We are faced with deep and radical fragmentation, as well as thoroughgoing confusion, if we try to think of what could be the reality that is treated by our physical laws...Both in relativity and in quantum theory the Cartesian order is leading to serious contradictions and confusions.

After an extensive analysis of the philosophical implications of quantum theory, Bohm concludes:

The explicate and manifest order of consciousness is not ultimately distinct from that of matter in general. Fundamentally these are essentially different aspects of the one overall order...The more comprehensive, deeper and more inward actuality is neither mind nor body but rather a yet higher-dimensional actuality, which is their common ground and which is of a nature beyond both...in which mind and body are ultimately one.[7]

Hence, for Bohm, the ultimate stuff of the universe must involve a synthesis of energy and consciousness.

Jantsch is the philosopher-spokesman for the evolutionary paradigm based on physicist Prigogine's Nobel Prize-winning work on dissipative structures. Jantsch describes ten unifying principles of evolution for this emerging paradigm of self-organization. Self-reference is the principle of relevance to Teilhard's ontology of panpsychism (all energy as consciousness):

Self-reference is the nondualistic principle *per se*. It implies self-organization without reference to any external authority...The basic unit of evolution is not a morphological structure, but a process structure...We may say that the *mind—* the dynamics of a system—is the basic evolutionary unit.[8]

Ramanand presents a cogent philosophical argument for the presence of consciousness in even the most basic physical energy in the universe.[9] Consciousness is present in every act of comprehension or perception. Consciousness has three aspects: cognition, conation, and affection. Reaction in an element is proof of congnition and hence of consciousness; and we have seen that even the most fundamental particles react to each other in terms of spin, charge, and mass. Conation is willing and acting. Affection is evidenced by self-modification, by a force acting upon itself (as in radioactive elements). Therefore, wherever we observe action, reaction, or self-modification, consciousness in at least a prototypical form is present. Thus, in the above context, Ramanand concludes, wherever there is energy, there must also be consciousness. The fact that Ramanand presents a modern expression of the most ancient Indian philosophy, the Vedic tradition, adds further depth and significance to Teilhard's ontological position.

In addition to this logical argument, there is a causal argument, cited frequently by Teilhard, for the panpsychic view of matter. That is, something cannot arise from nothing. It is logically absurd to suppose that the gamut of consciousness stops short below the level of life or mind. This would imply a discontinuity or lack of unity in the world that contradicts all our experience otherwise. Human consciousness can be nothing but a form of the universe's consciousness. Peirce, an early 20th-century American evolutionary idealist, argues that the human mind has developed under the same laws that govern the extramental realm; hence, it is only logical that reason think in accordance with nature's pattern.[10]

The argument of coherence is another powerful support for an idealist view of reality. By coherence, Teilhard does not mean only logical coherence in the traditional Hegelian sense. Teilhard's view explains more and is heuristically more powerful than a materialist view such as Monod's. An evolution of consciousness—of cognition, conation, and affection—explains the emergence of life and of man, and shows the direction of man's further evolution. The tendency toward increasing complexity, integration, and centricity of form is necessitated by the evolving consciousness. What appears to be a bewildering variety of form and structure—far beyond the needs of adaptation—becomes credible when the thread of an evolving consciousness is strung through the forms of this universe.

Huxley comments in his classic *Evolution in Action:*

> For a bioligist, much the easiest way is to think of mind and matter as two aspects of a single, underlying reality—shall we call it world-substance, the stuff out of which the world is made. At any rate, this fits more of the facts and leads to fewer contradictions than any other view.[11]

This is, for Huxley, the simplest way to explain the unique ability of mind to transmute quantity into quality, fact into sensation.

Similarly, Peirce finds the thesis that all matter is conscious attractive because of its ability to explain sensation. Mind/body dualism is unable to explain sensation. The "hylopathic" position Peirce takes maintains that the stimulus is of the same nature as the sensation it evokes, this nature being one of feeling, or consciousness.[12]

Glowienka discusses the Teilhardian concept of consciousness in matter from an Aristotelian point of view. He describes the pattern of the parts of material entities as being

inside of the parts thus patterned...Traditionally, this structuring, this patterning, in things, was given the name of "form"'...therefore, "material things" are
not exclusively "material"; they are also partially "spiritual."[13]

Glowienka suggests that all material things can be described as "conscious"
in the sense that their pattern is nonextended. A conscious being is defined
as one that can interiorize, as a nonextended part within itself, the very cause
of its relatedness to another. Again we see that sensation, or perception, is
taken to be the basis of consciousness, supporting Teilhard's connection between interiority and awareness.

Another aspect of Teilhard's ontology is its holism. As mentioned earlier,
this holism takes many forms. First, an attempt is made to include all aspects
of experience as data for interpretation. Second, the evolutionary process
itself involves a synthesis of ever more centered wholes. Third, each evolving center is potentially coextensive with the universe, and all are knit into
one grand unity through their mutual interactions and movement in the same
stream of becoming. Finally, the culmination of the evolution of human
centers will be their totalization into one organic whole. The first three points
will be critically analyzed in this section; the last will be considered in the
discussion of Teilhard's teleology.

Teilhard's attempt to synthesize multiple dimensions of experience into
his view has evoked strong reactions of both praise and criticism. Critics
generally maintain that science and philosophy, or objective and subjective
experience, are separate domains of investigation and that it is inappropriate
to mix them.[14] This assertion is based on the dualism of mind and matter,
nonextension and extension, established by Descartes, who maintained that
no interaction occurs between the two. The current philosophical trend,
however, is a call for precisely the sort of synthesis Teilhard attempts:

> This is the holistic view now seen as vital to balance the reductive method. The
> brain's ability to shift from its analytical left hemisphere to the integrative right
> hemisphere is often cited as an example. It...seeks a "new natural philosophy"
> based on organic and evolutionary principles.[15]

Whitehead, as mentioned in the historical review, was one of the early modern
philosophers who rejected the Cartesian bifurcation of matter and mind. In
discussing the philosophy of materialism, Whitehead suggests that we "conceive mental operations as among the factors which make up the constitu-
tion of nature"; and in terms of the holism of man, he says, "Let us ask
about our overwhelming persuasions as to our own personal body-mind relation. In the first place, there is the claim to unity. The human individual
is one fact, body and mind."[16]

Within the scientific community, also, the trend is toward a holistic view
of phenomena. Bohm asserts that both quantum theory and relativity theory
imply an "unbroken wholeness of the universe."[17] In a similar spirit, Huxley

observes "we have to ask how we can come to terms scientifically with a reality which combines both material and mental properties in its unitary pattern."[18]

Philosophically, an ontology that does not encompass all realms of experience cannot be complete. For Hegel and other rationalists, reason was the ultimate and highest mode of truth. They did not acknowledge the realm of mystical experience, of suprarational consciousness. For Teilhard, this realm was a living, experienced reality, as it has been for innumerable individuals. His philosophy, therefore, was impelled to include and incorporate this consciousness. The influence of mystical experience on Teilhard's ontological holism appears to be on his view of the essential unity of the universe.

The materialist philosopher will undoubtedly raise strong objections to this subjective avenue of obtaining knowledge. In fact, this is a basic difference between Monod and Teilhard. Monod's postulate of objectivity is closely related to the positivist criterion of verifiability, which maintains that only statements that can be verified by common sensory experience are acceptable as scientific knowledge.[19] This is a methodological criterion that should not dictate metaphysical conclusions. Science deals with one order of reality, that which can be perceived through the senses, and reaches is conclusions by the use of reason.

Ghosh, an Indian philosopher who, like Ramanand, has synthesized Western and Eastern experience, comments extensively on the issue of subjective versus objective knowledge:

> There are different orders of reality; the objective and physical is only one order...It is reasoned that to depart from the physical standard and the principle of personal or universal verification will lead to gross delusions and the admission of unverified truth and subjective fantasy into the realm of knowledge. But error and delusion and the introduction of personality and one's own subjectivity into the pursuit of knowledge are always present, and the physical or objective standards and methods do not exclude them.[20]

Similarly, Polanyi refers to the personal coefficient of the thinker, the "tacit dimension" of knowledge, and denies "that any participation of the knower in the shaping of knowledge must invalidate knowledge...Tacit knowing is in fact the dominant principle of all knowledge, and...its rejection would, therefore, automatically involve the rejection of any knowledge whatever."[21] Mystical experience, then, can and should be integrated into a truly holistic philosophy. It is a well-defined sphere of experience and has been documented in all cultures and eras.[22] Those who experience this consciousness unanimously maintain that it is more convincing than arguments based on sensory experience and reason.

According to Ramanand, mystical insight or "wisdom enables one to identify oneself with everything and every setting. Thus, there results an intimate knowledge, which is without the possibility of an error."[23] The limitations of reason and the human mind make objective knowledge vulnerable to error. Reason is based on the vagaries of the individual thinker, his environment, and his life experiences. Reason can also be strongly influenced by the thinker's physical and emotional state. The human senses can receive only a limited range of energy frequencies; furthermore, the same sensory stimuli do not lead to the same perceptions. Kant tells us how the rational mind organizes stimuli into perceptions and conceptions, according to preestablished categories. This is why Plato, Plotinus, Spinoza, Bergson, Whitehead, and others have maintained that intuition, a direct and synthetic vision, is a higher form of knowing. Mystical insight is one intuitive mode of knowing.

Teilhard's view of the evolutionary process as a synthesis of ever more centered wholes finds scientific as well as philosophical support. Certainly in the biological sphere this tendency is universally accepted. Harris describes the progression of evolution revealed by modern science as being toward an "increase in the integrity and indissolubility of the whole."[24] The central theme of Smut's evolutionary philosophy is the drive toward wholeness at all levels. Similarly, for Sellars the occurrence of creative synthesis through matter's inherent organizational properties generates an integrative causality in the universe. Leibniz and Whitehead conceive of a progressive integration of more complex and conscious wholes; Hegel, too, sees the becoming impelled by each unit's dialectical impulse to unite with its complement to form a more stable whole.

In addition to a holism of the evolutes, Teilhard's holism encompasses the totality of the universe. This relationship between the many and the one has been described in similar terms by many idealist philosophers—for example, Plotinus, Leibniz, Hegel, and Whitehead. Harris explains that modern scientific theory supports the wholeness, or unity, of the universe described by Teilhard.

> The scientific conspectus of the world is of a continuous process of activity progressively elaborating more complex and more highly integrated systems; yet the world itself, as a whole, is a totality systematically diversified and integrated in the same way... The entire structure is one of wholes, within wholes, within wholes, each expressing in its own character the general priniple of unity that is immanent throughout. (p. 454)

To summarize, Teilhard's ontology is based on the concept of centration, in which conscious energy, the basic stuff of the universe, is organized into increasingly centered, complex, and integrated wholes. This idealist view of energy as inherently conscious has been shown to be logically and scientifically valid and of value in providing continuity and coherence to the evolutionary process. The holism of Teilhard's evolutionary centration is also acceptable, being consistent with current scientific theory and numerous idealist philosophies. Teilhard's incorporation of the insights of mystical experience into his philosophy also contributes to the comprehensiveness and coherence of his ontological position.

CRITIQUE OF TEILHARD'S TELEOLOGY

Teilhard's teleology presents more philosophical problems than does his ontology. One reason for this is that his teleology is more ambiguous than the idealist oncology just discussed. In different essays and books, he handles the subject from many points of view. The concept of personalization has been chosen as the central teleological tenet for critical analysis in this study, for it appears to be a unifying theme among Teilhard's various approaches.

Again, mystical insight provides a strong influence in Teilhard's teleology. Teilhard believes that the evolutionary trend is toward an increase in the number of individuals who experience an ultrapersonalizing cosmic consciousness, not merely as a passing state, but as a permanent change in their awareness. Given the primary ontology that it is consciousness that is evolving, it is appropriate that the direction of evolution be described as a developmental change in awareness.

Certainly it is true that a great deal of attention is being directed toward "altered" states of consciousness. Cowling cites evidence from a number of sources indicating that the occurrence of mystical experience has been increasing in the last several decades.[25] Aurobindo and Ramanand also describe the direction of human evolution as being toward a supramental or wisdom consciousness that transcends three-dimensional, rational awareness, illuminating the unity of the universe. Again, it is noteworthy that Teilhard's view of evolution finds consonance with a number of tradtitions, Eastern as well as Western.

Whitehead also refers to "the ultimate unity of the multiplicity of actual fact with the primordial conceptual fact." He describes the perfection of the evolving entities of the universe as they are "completed by their everlasting union with their transformed selves, purged into conformation with the eternal order which is the final absolute 'wisdom.'"... Creativity achieves its supreme task of transforming disjoined multiplicity, with its diversities in contrast."[26] This teleology is comparable to Teilhard's idea of personalization through union, which is his teleological theme. This synthetic principle is evident in many areas of human experience. A union of parts into a whole does not result in a homogeneous mass. The parts are specialized and integrated into a harmony that sustains and supports each member. Individual organisms, as well as social units, illustrate this process. The trend toward mystical awareness and union is, then, a trend toward personalization. Union does, indeed, differentiate.

Teilhard's vision becomes less plausible when he speaks of the evolving union of mankind as the creation of a new organism. It is unclear whether he is speaking metaphorically or literally when he states that "mankind is more and more taking the form of an organism that possesses a physiology and, in the current phrase, a common 'metabolism' '' (*AE,* p. 36). The majority of his descriptions of totalization, however, are in terms of a transformation of consciousness:

> At present it seems inconceivable that persons should enter into contact through the depths of themselves...We must imagine for ourselves thinking molecules interiorized on one another when they reach their perfect conjunction. A perfect mutual transparency in a perfect self-possession. (*HE,* pp. 68–69)

This union of consciousness finds indicators in the formation of larger and larger social networks, parapsychological phenomena (such as telepathy) and, of course, the global communication systems now in operation.

Convergence as a state of universal consciousness appears to be occurring in the global phenomena Teilhard describes; convergence as a physiological phenomenon lacks any evidence. Teilhard's view of convergence as the final phase of evolution places a closure on the process that is unnecessary and undesirable. To deem mankind the last phase of earthly evolution exceeds the bounds of an appropriate anthropocentricity. There is no reason that consciousness should not continue to evolve into a suprahuman stage, and beyond.

Teilhard's placement of the driving force of evolution within the evolutes, innate in the conscious energy of the cosmos, saves him from the currently untenable position of supporting final causation, in the Aristotelian sense of the word. To review, final causation refers to a causal influence exerted by the end result of a process. Teleological explanation has traditionally been associated with this narrow conception, which has lost its status in modern philosophical circles.

However, the conception of a creative, immanent impulse toward self-transcendence, toward development into more complex and conscious entities, has received wide philosophical support. Spencer, Morgan, Alexander, Smuts, Bergson, Peirce, and Whitehead are among those who have postulated a similar potentiality existing in all forms of energy. This modern form of teleological explanation offers a view that can explain the directional movement of evolution without introducing logically problematic final causation. It also appears more satisfactory than Neo-Darwinian attempts to explain evolutionary progression solely on the basis of random mutations and natural selection. This is surely one of the mechanisms of evolution, but by itself it appears inadequate to explain the persistent directionality toward increasing complexity and consciousness.

The logic of Teilhard's argument for the irreversibility of human evolution is persuasive. To summarize, Teilhard maintains a universe that has produced self-awareness and a desire for immortality must be able to satisfy these needs; otherwise it would be structurally absurd. It is not clear, however, why he does not allow irreversibility to be a characteristic of all phases of evolution. The issue here is the meaning of death in Teilhard's teleology. Teilhard does not discuss what happens to the nonhuman evolute when it dies.

Death poses no problem in a materialistic view of evolution, which sees individual evolutes as transitory structures whose value is measured in terms of their reproductive success. Species and genes are the changeless entities, and even these change over time in response to selective pressures. In an idealistic view of evolution, however, death of the individual evolute can present a schematic difficulty. Consciousness, not structure, is evolving. If each prehuman center of conscious energy in Teilhard's scheme completely dissolves at its death, then there will be nothing remaining for the evolutionary forces to work with. The materialist has the genetic material available for natural selection; the idealist sees the gene as a manifestation of the whole, of the consciousness it is expressing. Therefore, there must be a consciousness, analogous to the gene, which survives the death of the individual and which is subject to the gradual evolutionary change expressed by the gene.

Idealist philosophers who have constructed systems similar to Teilhard's have utilized the concept of reincarnation, or metempsychosis, to solve the problem of death in an evolving consciousness. Leibniz described a process of metamorphosis, and would not allow the evolving soul-monads to entirely quit their physical bodies and pass into completely new ones. Ramanand also discusses a process of reincarnation that is consistent with current theories of evolution. Briefly, among the nonhuman evolutes, it is a group-consciousness (the species) that is the unit of evolution, and the gene is its physical unit of expression. Natural selection and survival of the fittest are operative principles of evolutionary development in the group-consciousness. As differentiation increases with evolution, the individual conscious energy becomes the unit of evolution. The individual human units of conscious energy are evolving into higher levels of consciousness, gathering experiences that promote this evolution through the succession of physical bodies.

CONCLUSION

Teilhard's idealist philosophy of evolution resolves several of the problems that materialism is unable to dispel. Through the underlying ontology of conscious energy, having an innate tendency to evolve, the continuity of evolution is maintained despite the emergence of new levels of existence. Teilhard's holistic ontology is another of distinctive and valuable qualities. The individual evolute and the entire becoming are considered in all their aspects and modes of experience, synthesized into an organic unity. Acknowledgment of the validity of mystical experience and the insights it offers is another strength of Teilhard's worldview, a strength that is rarely found in Western philosophical systems. Teilhard's vision of an evolutionary development of consciousness portends an increasing knowledge and wisdom as mankind's evolutionary, self-transcending future—not an arbitrary ethical choice, such as that which Monod offers as man's future.

The weakness of the Teilhardian vision is related to his conceptions of convergence and death. These are aspects of Teilhard's philosophy that are not entirely typical of idealist philosophies, and need not be considered essential for an idealist metaphysic. It is, however, true that many Western idealistic systems place limits on the future possibilities of evolutionary development; for example, Hegel and the rationalists saw reason as the final culmination of natural process. Given the contemporary view of an ever-changing, even expanding, universe, these systems must be revised. Teilhard's concept of convergence, although it postulates a suprarational awareness as its outcome, must also be rejected for its imposition of a closed end to what appears to be a limitless evolutionary potential in conscious energy.

REFERENCES

1. Pierre Teilhard de Chardin, *Human Energy,* trans. R. Hague (New York: Harcourt Brace Jovanovich, 1969), p. 20; hereafter cited in the text as *HE.*

2. Pierre Teilhard de Chardin, *Activation of Energy,* trans. R. Hague (London: William Collins Sons Ltd., 1970), p. 30; hereafter cited in the text as *AE.*

3. H. H. Price, *"Clarity is Not Enough,"* *Proceedings of the Aristotelian Society,* Supp. Vol. XIX (1945), 3-9, 20-30; rpt. in *Contemporary Philosophic Problems,* ed. Y. H. Krikorian and A. Edel (New York: Macmillan, 1959).

4. Erich Jantsch, "Unifying Principles of Evolution," in *The Evolutionary Vision,* ed. E. Jantsch, AAAS Selected Symposia Series, 61 (Boulder, CO: Westview, 1981), p. 85.

5. Jantsch, "Unifying Principles of Evolution," p. 91.

6. Bernhard Rensch, *Biophilosophy,* trans. C. A. M. Sym (New York: Columbia University Press, 1971), p. 270.

7. David Bohm, *Wholeness and the Implicate Order* (London: Routledge & Kegan Paul, 1980), pp. xiii-vv, 208-209.

8. Jantsch, "Unifying Principles of Evolution," pp. 89-90.

9. S. Ramanand, *Evolutionary Spiritualism* (Bisalpur, India: Sahu Kashinath Mittal, Sadhana Karyalaya, 1956), p. 46.

10. Peter T. Turley, *Peirce's Cosmology* (New York: Philosophical Library, 1977), p. 81

11. Julian Huxley, *Evolution in Action* (1953; rpt. New York: Harper, 1966), p. 77.

12. Turley, p. 80.

13. Emerine Glowienka, "Notes on Consciousness in Matter," *New Scholasticism,* 43 (1969), pp. 602-13.

14. Alfred P. Stiernotte, "An Interpretation of Teilhard as Reflected in Recent Literature," *Zygon,* 3 (1968), pp. 377-425.

15. Arthur Fabel, *Cosmic Genesis,* Teilhard Studies Number 5 (Chambersburg, PA: Anima Books, 1981), pp. 1-2.

16. Alfred North Whitehead, *Modes of Thought* (1938; rpt. New York: Capricorn Books, 1958), pp. 214, 218.

17. *Wholeness and the Implicate Order,* p. xv.

18. *Evolution in Action,* p. 30.

19. Alfred Jules Ayer, *Language, Truth and Logic* (1936; rpt. New York: Dover, 1946).

20. Aurobindo Ghosh, *The Life Divine,* 3 ed. (New York: India Library Society, 1965), p. 580.

21. Michael Polanyi, *The Study of Man* (Chicago: University of Chicago Press, 1959), p. 13.

22. F. C. Happold, *Mysticism,* 2 ed. (London: Penguin, 1967); Walter T. Stace, *The Teachings of the Mystics* (New York: Mentor Books, New American Library, 1960); Evelyn Underhill, *Mysticism,* 12 ed. (1910; rpt. Cleveland: Meridian Books, World Publishing Co., 1970).

23. *Evolutionary Spiritualism,* p. 100.

24. Errol E. Harris, *The Foundations of Metaphysics in Science* (1965; rpt. Lanham, MD: University Press of America, 1983), p. 455.

25. Richard Cowling, "The Relationship of Mystical Experience, Differentiation and Creativity in College Students," Diss., New York University, 1982, p. 12.

26. Alfred North Whitehead, *Process and Reality* (1929; rpt. New York: Harper, 1960), pp. 525-28.

5

ROGERS'S EVOLUTIONARY MODEL

INTRODUCTION

Martha E. Rogers, currently professor emeritus at New York University in the Division of Nursing, presented an evolutionary model of man to the nursing profession in 1970 with the publication of *Theoretical Basis of Nursing.*[1] No other conceptual model for nursing has evoked so much controversy, for it was in clear contradistinction to all the nursing theories in use at that time, and remains so today. Rogers has continually refined and elaborated the model, in conjunction with numerous empirical research studies designed to test hypotheses derived from it, and also in connection with an undergraduate and master's educational curriculum designed to allow students to apply the model to clinical practice.

Dr. Rogers has published several articles since 1970 explicating her model of unitary human beings, and she is completing a new book that presents extensive revisions and refinements of the original work. For this reason, the description of the model presented in this chapter, and its analysis in later chapters, is based extensively on a set of personal interviews with Rogers, as well as on the original book and later articles. Transcripts of these interviews are included in the appendix of this study.

Rogers's outlook is based on the most recent theories in the physical and biological sciences, and on the attempts of some contemporary philosophers

59

to include these insights into a coherent worldview. It is a unique synthesis of current knowledge into a model whose primary focus is man as an evolving being. In her early work, Rogers presents a historical backdrop for her model, describing the developments in philosophy and science that led to the Cartesian and Newtonian worldviews. "The rise of modern science with its emphasis on a mechanistic approach and mind-body dualism was a firm denial of man and nature as a single system." However, Rogers maintains, "the introduction of evolutionary theory and the discrediting of the theory of spontaneous generation in the latter half of the 19th century cracked the veneer of man's belief in his separate existence" (*TBN*, p. 29). Einstein's theory of relativity and field theory further shook the old philosophical edifice. The basic outlook, then, from which Rogers built her model was as follows: "Man is a unified phenomenon subject to natural laws . . . . Man's consciousness and creativity are integral dimensions of man's wholeness" (*TBN*, p. 34). A general summary of the model will first be provided, followed by a detailed description of the concepts of particular concern to this study—the human energy field and the principle of helicy.

ROGERS'S CONCEPTUAL MODEL OF UNITARY HUMAN BEINGS— GENERAL DESCRIPTION

The structural elements of Rogers's model include definitions, four building blocks, or postulates, which are accepted as basic assumptions, three principles of homeodynamics, and a delineation of some correlates of human patterning. Since Rogers's definitions of man and environment involve a language of specificity, with several unique meanings, terms relevant to the ensuing discussion are presented below:[2]

- **Energy field**—the fundamental unit of the living and nonliving. Field is a unifying concept. Energy signifies the dynamic nature of the field. Energy fields are infinite.

- **Pattern**—the distinguishing characteristic of an energy field perceived as a single wave.

- **Four-dimensional**—a nonlinear domain without spatial or temporal attributes.

- **Unitary man (human field)**—an irreducible, four-dimensional energy field identified by pattern and manifesting characteristics that are specific to the whole and that cannot be predicted from knowledge of the parts.

- **Environment (environmental field)**—an irreducible, four-dimensional energy field identified by pattern and integral with the human field.

Rogers describes a universe of open systems that is inherently negentropic and characterized by continual change. Man and environment, then, are open systems, are infinite, and are integral with each other; that is, they are complementary, and their boundaries are imaginary and arbitrary. Reality—the universe, and all within it—is four-dimensional; space and time are man-made concepts based on linear Euclidean geometric notions. Since Rogers's concept of the human energy field and of evolution will be extensively discussed later in this chapter, the postulates, principles and correlates of the model will now be described.

Postulates

Energy fields. Energy fields are the fundamental units of the universe. The words "energy" and "field" are used in the general language sense, not as they are used in particular branches of science, such as physics or biology. " 'Field' is a unifying concept; 'energy' signifies it is dynamic; energy fields are infinite; so these are really infinite dynamic unities." [3] When an energy field is assigned its arbitrary boundary, it must be taken as an irreducible whole, with characteristics relating to the whole rather than to any of its parts. Rogers contrasts her view of holism to the less radical, more "popular usage of the term 'holistic' generally signifying a summation of parts." [4]

In the early book, Rogers described the energy field as being electrical in nature. This, however, is not her present view. The energy field is four-dimensional, identified by its pattern, and electrical phenomena are a manifestation of pattern. Rogers's use of the term "energy" apparently implies a state of continuous motion or change, the dynamic nature of the field.

Openness. The postulate of openness affirms that man exists in a universe of open systems; in fact, there are no closed systems. She expressly rejects the closed-system mechanics of Newtonian physics, and along with it such concepts as equilibrium and adaptation. The openness of energy fields implies two distinct characteristics. First, the human and environmental fields are in continual and simultaneous interaction with each other, in a noncausal relationship. Second, open systems are negentropic; they are always in a process of transformation into "increasing heterogeneity, differentiation, diversity, complexity of pattern." [5] The universe as a whole is also negentropic, contradictory to the old entropic model of a universe running down into homogeneity.

Pattern. Pattern is an assumption that is gaining increasing importance in Rogers's model as it undergoes further elaboration and testing. Pattern identifies and is unique to each energy field. All the characteristics and behaviors of any field are manifestations of pattern, and it is these manifestations that are changing in the process of evolution. Pattern is perceived as a single wave; that is, it manifests and is apprehended as a whole. Since pattern is continually changing, the life process appears to be a dance of rhythmical waves vibrating at various frequencies. Pattern constitutes the

il nature of an energy field (PI, 1). It is not to be equated with structure of any physical phenomenon, for it continues even beyond death.

Four-Dimensionality. Four-dimensionality has proven to be the most difficult postulate for readers to understand in Rogers's model. Reality is
nonlinear, nontemporal, nonspatial. Rogers maintains that this is not only
a description of what reality is not. Nonlinearity means that reality "spreads
all over; it's not a line"; it represents an infinite, transcendent domain.
Nonspatial means it "cannot be bound in spatial geometry," and nontemporal refers to the relativity of time and to the "relative present" for a given
individual.[6] Paranormal phenomena, such as precognition, telepathy, reincarnation, and meditative modalities, which indicate an awareness "beyond
waking," can be explained by the postulate of four-dimensionality.

Rogers emphasizes that all four of these assumptions must be synthesized
to form the basis of her conceptual model of unitary human beings. Out
of this synthesis emerge the principles of homeodynamics. These principles
describe the nature and direction of evolution, and the correlates of patterning, which identify some expected manifestations of evolving human field
patterns. A synthetic summary of the four postulates into one sentence may
take the following form: The fundamental unit of the universe is the energy
field, which is an irreducible, infinite, dynamic, open, four-dimensional unity,
integral with the environment and identified by pattern.

Principles of Homeodynamics

The principle of resonancy describes "the continuous change from lower
to higher frequency wave patterns in the human and environmental fields."[7]
As mentioned before, the waves referred to here are not the electromagnetic
waves of physics or any other specific discipline. Rogers emphasizes that it
is pattern that should be the focus in this principle, not wave. "Higher frequency" refers to the acceleration in the rate of change in patterning that
is occurring. "I use . . . frequency and wave as general language to get across
the idea of nonrepeating rhythmicities and acceleration" (PI, 1). Rogers por-
trays the life process in man as a symphony of rhythmical vibrations
oscillating at various frequencies. The overall pattern of the human field is
"a wave phenomenon encompassing man in his entirety" (*TBN*, p. 101).

The principle of helicy postulates that evolution is a process of continuous,
innovative, probabilistic, increasing diversity of human and environmental
field patterns characterized by nonrepeating rhythmicities. This principle will
be elaborated later in this chapter, as it is the tenet that describes the nature
and direction of change in the evolutionary process.

The principle of integrality rejects causality in the universe, accepting only the "continuous, mutual human field and environmental field process."[8]
Mechanistic and deterministic explanations of events have no place in this

model. "The appearance of causality does not make it so. In a universe of open systems mutual simultaneity is explicit. That is, man and environment change together."[9] Rogers derived the principle of noncausality from the theories of modern physics; she specifically cites Heisenberg's principle of uncertainity, quantum theory, and Einstein's theory of relativity. She also calls upon Russell's rejection of causality for support of this view. Rogers rejects the old causal view of man adapting to the environment.

Correlates of Patterning

The indices, or correlates, of patterning are attempts to predict the nature of the increasing diversity and higher frequency of field pattern that is seen as individuals evolve. Rogers does not identify changes that occur in the human species as a group; her focus is the individual. Therefore, the relative nature of the correlates of patterning is evident. Rogers formerly used the term "indices of development," but has recently rejected this term because it implies a linear progression of patterns. She is in the process of revising the postulated correlates, but is certain to include three sets: (1) from pragmatic to imaginary to visionary, (2) from sleeping to waking to beyond waking, and (3) from materiality to ethereality. Rogers clarified in an interview that the proper way to interpret these correlates is that they are "experienced as"; that is the individual manifesting higher-frequency wave patterning would experience (and be experienced as) visionary, ethereal, or beyond waking manifestations (PI, 2). These correlates will be discussed further in connection with the principle of helicy.

ROGERS'S OVERALL VIEW OF EVOLUTION

For Rogers, evolution is a creative, innovative becoming characterized by continuous repatterning of energy fields. In a four-dimensional reality, evolution cannot be described as a temporal or linear progression, but it does display the trend inherent in all open systems—that of negentropy. The evolutionary emergence of new patterns allows for the actualization of the rich potentialities for self-transcendence inherent in all energy fields. Human field repatterning occurs in the mutual man/environment process.

Rogers explicitly rejects a hierarchical view of the evolutionary process. In her earlier book, Rogers viewed man as standing at the pinnacle of the becoming, and emphasized man's unique qualities of sentience, thought, and feeling. However, from the interviews, it appears that these conceptions are revised:

> I'm not going to talk about man being at the peak of anything; I don't know
> whether he is or not. We're pretty conceited—but we are different . . . . Com-
> parative dissertations between man and other animals, and between life and nonlife,
> I'll leave to somebody else . . . . I think that they try to do it on gross observa-
> tion, not on any kind of depth thinking. (PI, 1)

Rogers now prefers to focus on man's evolutionary potentials, without implying that they are unique or higher than those of other life forms; "so it
will be, what are man's capacities, not whether these are like or different
from . . . . The fact that there may be many other things with similar potentials is great. There are. But that does not happen to be the primary concern
of nursing" (PI, 2).

Rogers's conception of evolution does not focus on physical evolution,
species, or genes. As mentioned before, "pattern" does not refer to structure or other visible forms. Evolution is a process of change toward higher-
frequency wave patterns and increasing diversity of patterns in the human
and environmental fields. The emphasis is on the individual human field,
although Rogers frequently refers to man in the general sense and to the evolutionary implications of accelerating cultural change:

> Man's advent into outer space made explicit this new world. Escalating science
> and technology help to underwrite new paradigms and to hasten the ending of
> the industrial age. Noise, confusion, and insecurities mount as the speed of change
> crescendos. Old values lie moribund among the detritus of famous last words.
> Man moves to transcend himself.[10]

The concept of natural selection is contradicted in the open-systems, noncausal worldview Rogers proposes. Adaptation and randomness are both excluded. Adaptation implies one energy fireld being causally influenced by
an environment, and is replaced by the concept of mutual process, or the
principle of integrality. Man and environment change together. Rogers does
not believe that the future manifestations of pattern can be predicted, but
she does maintain that knowledgeable guesses can be made; in other words,
evolution is probabilistic. "I don't think that it is randomness, in the sense
that I think the term is commonly used" (PI, 1). She admits that evolution
is an orderly process, but it is innovative and creative, so that "maybe we're
going to find a lot of paradoxes in what we think is order. And some of
the things, maybe as we know more, that we think look chaotic, are not
chaotic" (PI, 1).

Rogers believes that consciousness—in a very global sense of he word—is
rudimentary throughout the universe (PI, 1). However, she avoids "consciousness," because it has so many different meanings. "Awareness" is the
term she prefers, and also uses "perception", to indicate manifestations of
pattern characterized by sentience. A number of the correlates of patterning

relate to changes in awareness that occur as manifestations of increasingly diverse and higher-frequency patterning—for example, perceptions of time passing, awareness of one's own field motion, sleep/wake and meditative modalities, and imaginative/visionary qualities. The evolution of consciousness is an integral aspect of human field patterning;

> Coming into awareness is postulated to represent new levels of complexity with correlates in the ongoing development of cognition and feelings. The capacity to experience one's self and the world and to make sense out of one's experience is an emergent. (*TBN*, p.93).

A final aspect of Rogers's overall view of evolution should be mentioned before we turn to the specific tenets to be analyzed in this study. This is the theory of accelerating evolution. The higher-frequency wave patterns signify an acceleration in the rate of change of the field. Rogers cites numerous instances of the acceleration of change in human society and environmental fields; this is common sociological knowledge. On the individual level, too, an acceleration of change is postulated, for man and environment evolve together. Higher-frequency wave patterns and more complex forms change more rapidly. Accelerating human field rhythms are coordinate with higher-frequency environmental field patterns.

THE HUMAN ENERGY FIELD

Rogers's conception of the human energy field has been selected as the element in which the ontological implications of her view will most likely be found. In the chapter, only Rogers's descriptions will be presented; the next chapter contains an analysis of the ontology implicit in this delineation of the human energy field.

Unitary man, or the human field, is defined as an irreducible, four-dimensional energy field indentified by pattern. According to Rogers, the physical body does not constitute the human being. In fact, field patterning is continuous "and is not determined by something called death or nondeath, or by living or nonliving" (PI, 2). Every human field is unique, because its pattern is unique and its environment is unique.

The human energy field is synergistic; that is, it has characteristics that are derived from the whole and cannot be predicted from the parts taken separately. Rogers explicitly rejects all dualistic conceptions of man. "The mind-matter dualism of Cartesian philosophy continues to mitigate against a conception of man's unity" (*TBN*, p. 45).

The energy field is four-dimensional, so that physicalistic characterizations of it as being electrical, electromagnetic, or chemical in nature are unsuitable. "Energy" is used to signify the ever-changing, dynamic, nonmaterial nature of the human field. When questioned as to the nature of human energy, Rogers responded, "Pattern" (PI, 1). Pattern itself is ever changing, and is perceived through its manifestations.

The manifestations of pattern are wave phenomena, which are displayed by the field as a whole. In her description of the human energy field, Rogers emphasizes such manifestations as self awareness, emotions, and rational thought. Personality is also a manifestation of human field patterning. Rogers characterizes her model as humanistic, in the sense that unitary man has the capacity to knowingly participate in the evolutionary process. "Abstraction and imagery, language and thought, sensation and emotion are fundamental attributes of man's humanness" (*TBN*, p. 67)

Unitary man is a field of resonating waves, or rhythmical vibrations. The rhythmicities of the human field are nonrepeating and ever changing, but they do allow for probabilistic predictions to be made. Patterns do not repeat themselves, but similarities in successive waves allow for continuity of the field to be maintained. What is commonly called the process of human development is explainable in terms of these nonrepeating rhythmicities. Rogers prefers to avoid the term "development," because of its connotations of linearity and temporality. However, she describes the orderliness of man's becoming as involving creative, negentropic wave patterns of greater diversity and higher frequency. Rogers rejects developmental norms, because change is relative, but she does emphasize manifestations of repatterning that are related to human perceptual capacities or, to use the preferable term, man's evolving awareness. This will be discussed further in connection with the principle of helicy.

Although Rogers insists that the human field is infinite, with only imaginary boundaries, she accepts the necessity of arbitrarily delineating boundaries on a pragmatic level, and holds the unique pattern of the individual field to be of primary importance. She does not dismiss as illusory, the individual sense of self; rather, views this as manifestation of pattern. Evolution, however, is a process of self-transcendence by the human field:

> Man's capacity for experiencing himself and his world identifies his humanness. Abstract thought couched in language enables him to grope toward cosmic understanding. The arts and sciences, philosophy and religion attest to man's evolutionary potential with transcendence of his present self. (*TBN*, p. 73)

PRINCIPLE OF HELICY

The principle of helicy describes the nature and direction of change in the human and environmental fields. It depicts "the continuous, innovative, probabilistic, increasing diversity of human and environmental field patterns characterized by nonrepeating rhythmicities."[11] In her early book, Rogers stated that this principle postulates the evolutionary emergence of cognition and feelings in the human field; this appears to be, at least in part, what the current definition refers to. This will be made clear by examining the correlates of patterning, which are based on the principle of helicy.

The correlates of patterning describe the evolution of unitary human beings from lesser to greater diversity, and from longer to shorter rhythms. Rogers explained in an interview that these correlates should be considered as changes that are "experienced as" by the individual. For example, less diverse field patterning would mean the individual experiences time as passing slowly, whereas more diverse patterning would manifest time experienced as racing, or as seeming continuous. Less diverse human field motion is experienced as a slower, more diverse as faster. Less diverse field patterning is experienced as pragmatic, material, or manifesting sleep; more diverse is experienced as visionary, ethereal, or beyond waking.

Many students of Rogers's model have misconstrued the above correlates as describing an evolution of the human field into a four-dimensional awareness. Rogers specifically addressed this issue in an interview, and made it clear that this is not a correct interpretation. All human fields—all reality, in fact— are four-dimensional. The above correlates signify evolution from longer-wave, lower-frequency, less diverse manifestation of field pattern into shorter-wave, higher-frequency, more diverse manifestations. They may signify an evolution of awareness, or perceptual evolution, but four-dimensionality is a given; it is the very nature of the human field, regardless of its mode of awareness. (PI, 2)

Rogers uses the term "diversity" in the general language sense. A synonym for diversity is variety. In her early book, in addition to diversity, Rogers described the direction of evolution as being toward increasing complexity, differentiation, and heterogeneity. In an interview, Rogers explains that this change in terminology does not represent a substantive change in the principle of helicy, but rather is a semantic change. She feels that the other terms mentioned above were being misinterpreted, leading to much ambiguity and confusion. She explained that in a universe of open systems, by definition all energy fields are evolving into increasing complexity, differentiation, and heterogeneity. The reason for the choice of "diversity" to describe the direction of evolution "was to stick to one word that, hopefully, would be less confusing" (PI, 2).

Another issue Rogers addressed in interviews was that of how a direction for evolution could occur in a noncausal universe. It appears that the answer to this query lies in the very nature of open systems. Their innate tendency is negentropic, and negentropy is change in a specific direction, not caused by any outside agency, but by the very nature of the system.

The negentropic nature of the human field explains how evolution can be a continually creative and innovative process, while at the same time allowing for probabilistic predictions to be made with reasonable success. There are numerous potentialities inherent in any human energy field, not all of which are actualized. The potentialities are due to the inherently negentropic, self-transcending qualities of an open system. The creativity and spontaneity are due to the fact that changes emerge out of the interaction process between the human and environmental fields—not from any previous or future determinants.

"Nonrepeating rhythmicities" also are an aspect of the principle of helicy, and are related to the probabilistic nature of evolutionary change. Rhythms are series of wave patterns that are similar, but not identical. The fact that the human field evolves rhythmically, therefore, makes it possible to posit knowledgeable guesses about the direction of evolutionary change for a particular individual. The human field rhythms may be in or out of harmony with the environmental rhythms, but they are always interacting with each other and changing together. Hence, both human and environmental rhythms are accelerating in their rate of oscillation in the current century, and will continue to do so.

SUMMARY

The view of evolution Rogers proposed is of a continually innovative repatterning of energy fields—a negentropic, self-transcending process characterized by accelerating rhythms and increasing diversity of the evolutes. Evolution occurs in a nonlinear, nonspatial, nontemporal matrix, a four-dimensional reality in which causality is an illusion. The evolutes, energy fields, are infinite and integral with an infinite environment. Energy fields are open systems, permeating and permeated by their environmental fields, identified and distinguished by their unique but ever changing rhythmic patterns. The human energy field is characterized by a conscious awareness of and the capacity for knowing participation in this universal becoming.

REFERENCES

1. *An Introduction of the Theoretical Basis of Nursing* (Philadelphia: F.A. Davis, 1970) hereafter cited in the text as *TBN.*

2. Revised definitions, dated November 22, 1982.

3. Personal interview with Rogers, December 12, 1983; hereafter cited in the test as PI, 1.

4. Martha E. Rogers, "Science of Unitary Human Beings: A Paradigm for Nursing," in *Family Health: A Theoretical Approach to Nursing Care,* ed. I.W. Clements and F.B. Roberts (New York: Wiley, 1983), p. 1 of article.

5. "Science of Unitary Human Beings," Glossary.

6. Personal interview with Rogers, January 31, 1984; hereafter cited in the text as PI, 2.

7. "Science of Unitary Human Beings," p. 2 of article.

8. "Science of Unitary Human Beings," p. 3 of article.

9. Martha E. Rogers, "Nursing: A Science of Unitary Man," in *Conceptual Models for Nursing Practice,* ed. J.P. Riehl and C. Roy, 2 ed. (New York: Appleton-Century-Crofts, 1980), p. 5 of article.

10. Martha E. Rogers, "Beyond the Horizon," in *The Nursing Profession: A Time to Speak* (New York: McGraw, 1982), p. 1 of article.

11. Revised definitions, dated November 22, 1982.

METAPHYSICAL IMPLICATIONS
OF ROGERS'S MODEL

INTRODUCTION

The purpose of the historical review of evolutionary thought and the critical analyses of the philosophies of Monod and Teilhard was to present the numerous metaphysical issues involved in the concept of evolution—specifically, those issues relating to the ontology and teleology of evolution. Toward the goal of providing a deeper understanding of the evolutionary nursing model Rogers developed, the ways in which some prominent philosphers have dealt with these issues were reviewed, and the antithetical views of Monod and Teilhard were critiqued in depth. At this point, it may be helpful to summarize some of the main ontological and teleological issues that the evolutionary philosophers previously examined have dealt with. After this has been done, the views of Rogers presented in the previous chapter will be analyzed for their explicit, as well as implicit, positions in relation to the identified issues.

Russell provides a concise and accurate account of the issues with which all the philosophers of evolution have struggled:

There are many questions—and among them those that are of the profoundest
interest to our spiritual life . . . . Has the universe any unity of plan or purpose,
or is it a fortuitous concourse of atoms? Is consciousness a permanent part of
the universe, giving hope of indefinite growth in wisdom, or is it a transitory ac-
cident on a small planet on which life must ultimately become impossible[1]

The first question Russell poses relates to teleology, the second to ontology,
in evolutionary philosophy. Within these two general philosophical questions,
several subquestions can be derived that identify the particular issues involved.
Some of the ontological questions addressed in the previous pages are, What
is evolving? What is its essential nature—can it be reduced to smaller units,
or is it an irreducible whole? What is the relationship between an evolute
and the rest of the universe? How is the continuity of the evolute or of evolution maintained? What is the role of death in the evolutionary process? The
teleological aspects of evolution involve such questions as, How do seemingly new properties, such as life and the human mind, emerge? Is there a
consistent direction to the evolutionary process? Does this direction imply
a purpose or meaning to evolution? Is evolution a creative or a mechanical
process? For each of these questions, I will attempt to identify the implied
or explicit answers provided by Rogers's conceptual model, drawing upon
the insights gained from the historical review and the analyses of Monod
and Teilhard.

ONTOLOGICAL IMPLICATIONS OF ROGERS'S MANUAL

In Rogers's conceptual system, the energy field is held to be the fundamental unit of the universe. Energy fields are open systems, in constant change,
and can therefore be identified as the evolute in a Rogerian ontology. Rogers's
concept of the energy field is somewhat analogous to Teilhard's psychic
center, which represents his evolutionary unit and which also consists of
energy of a metaphysical sort. Neither Rogers nor Teilhard uses the term
"energy" in the narrow meaning of physics. Rogers's energy fields are four-
dimensional and nonmaterial; Teilhard's centers are composed of conscious
energy, characterized by immanence or interiority. "Energy" for Rogers
implies continuous, dynamic activity. Teilhard takes this one step further,
claiming that this activity implies a rudimentary consciousness. As chapter
4 showed, Rogers does consider consciousness to be fundamental in the
universe, and given her acquaintance with the philosophical implication of
modern physics as discussed in chapter 3, Teilhard's delineation of energy
as being psychic in nature does not appear contradictory to her model. [2]
A closer examination of the implications of "pattern" in Rogers's model
may help to clarify the suggestion that her energy fields are characterized
by an elemental consciousness or subjectivity. Pattern is what identifies each

energy field, and it is unique to each field; Rogers describes it as the essence of the field. This can be called the subjectivity of the field, using the following meanings of the term "subjective": "of or relating to the essential being of that which supports attributes or relations; peculiar to a particular individual; personal."[3] Pattern is not any material structure or phenomenon; yet, all behaviors, qualities, and characteristics of the field are manifestations of pattern.

Whitehead's conception of "subjective aim" may help to further explore the ontological possibilities of a four-dimensional field pattern that can manifest reason, feelings, and awareness. For Whitehead, every actual entity is a throb of emotion, a process of becoming for the satisfaction of its subjective aim. Subjective aim is the unifying focus of all the feelings experienced by the actual occasions. There is no vacuous actuality, no entity devoid of subjective immediacy; subjective aim guides—or patterns—the becoming of an actual occasion. Of course, Rogers would not agree with the causal nature of this view; but the attempt here is to suggest an analogy that may enhance the meaning of Rogers's ontological unit, an energy field identified by pattern. In this analogy, pattern is being compared with subjective aim.

Rogers specifically rejects the suggestion that pattern is analogous to Aristotle's form because Aristotle's system is causal (PI, 2). However, pattern as an internal nonmaterial organizing and unifying design can very loosely be described as "form." In her early book, Rogers stated that the energy field imposes pattern on its parts. Her more recent view of pattern does not appear to incorporate this deterministic relationship. Pattern is the distinguishing characteristic of an energy field, and all of the field's attributes are manifestions of its pattern, which is itself continually changing in successive rhythmic waves.

Since all reality for Rogers is four-dimensional, an analysis of four-dimensionality may aid in further understanding the nature of the energy field. Rogers makes the point that the " 'human field' and 'relative present' are identical."[4] Again the element of subjectivity is apparent, for the perception of time is a subjective experience. One is reminded here of Bergson's concept of time as *durée*. the continuous flow of conscious experience.[5] Like Rogers, Bergson rejects the reality of space and linear time, viewing them as creations of the human intellect out of pragmatic necessity. Similarly, Rogers comments, "There is no space or time in this system. All those are man-made concepts . . . . It's just something that gets us . . . . to some meals on time" (PI, 1). If the human energy field is a nonspatial, nontemporal, and nonlinear entity, yet identified by a unique and personal subjectivity (pattern), one is tempted to describe it as a center of conscious energy, as Teilhard has done.

Jantsch's description of the evolutionary principle of self-reference, as mentioned in chapter 3, may also aid in illuminating the metaphysical potentialities of Rogers's concept of the human energy field. To review, self-reference refers to self-organization, implying "mind" in the dynamics of a system. Perhaps, then, Rogers's pattern can be seen as a principle of self-organization or mind, in a very general sense, that is unique to every energy field.

Most of the evolutionary philosophers discussed in this study have addressed the issue of holism. Rogers specifically rejects the reductionist viewpoint represented by Monod. Energy fields are irreducible. The teleonomic structure of Monod, which functions as a unity, is not characterized by wholeness in the sense of irreducibility. Indeed, Monod's major thesis is that the teleonomic apparatus is reducible to the interactions of proteins and completely determined by the genetic material. In Rogers's human energy field, proteins and genes have no role. The field's characteristics are specific to the whole.

Rogers's holism is similar in two respects to Teilhard's holism. They both include all aspects of human experience as basis for their descriptions of the qualities and potentialities of their evolute. The within and the without, subjectivity and objectivity, are considered. Mystical experience, paranormal phenomena, emotions, as well as scientific data, are synthesized in their ontological views.

Another aspect of holism shared by both Rogers and Teilhard is the monistic perspective of each evolute's being related to the entire universe. This aspect or Rogers's holism is more extreme than Teilhard's, for she maintains that individual boundaries are imaginary and that the energy field is integral with the environment. Nevertheless, every energy field is identified by a unique pattern, which implies that it has a personal, ontological reality. This is the familiar philosophical paradox of the one versus the many. Philosophers who have attempted to reconcile these two aspects of reality, rather than accepting only one as real, somethimes refer to the concept of the "concrete universal" to explain this seeming contradiction.[6] Teilhard's thought takes this form in a pluralistic monadism.

Rogers's referrals to meditative modalities and their manifestations of cosmic consciousness seem to imply that she does acknowledge the ultimate unity, or wholeness, of the universe. The universe is a "patterned wholeness." Energy fields are infinite, with arbitrarily delineated boundaries, and they are integral with their environment, which is the remainder of the universe. The affinities with Teilhard, as well as with other monistic philosophers, appear quite strong. The element of continuous change is unusual, however, in monistic worldviews. Bergson is a notable exception. For him, the *élan vital* is the one substance of the world, and is the continuously moving, creative process of life.

Rogers's model does not directly suggest a progressive integration or centration into increasingly organic wholes, as is seen in Teihard's ontology. However, the concept of open systems implies a drive toward heterogeneity, differentiation, and complexity. Integration is the natural accompaniment of these qualities. More complex systems must be more highly integrated. Biologically, this rule can easily be demonstrated. Whitehead's process philosophy also proposes the progressive self-organization and integration of actual entities. Monod, too, recognizes this basic trend in evolving teleonomic systems.

Closely related to conceptions of the wholeness, or unity, of the universe is the relationship between the evolute and its environment. In this matter, Rogers's view diverges from those of both Monod and Teilhard, who see this relationship as being rather one-sided. Monod sees the evolute adapting to its environment, and Teilhard emphasizes the intercentric relationships among the evolutes rather than between the evolute and its environment. Rogers's view of the integrality of man and environment, their constant mutual interaction and penetration, goes beyond that of most Western philosophers. Rogers stated in an interview that Eastern philophies have major similarities with her model; "certainly they have a sense of integralness, I think, that transcends the Wester view" (PI, 2). Change occurs through the mutual man/environment process. This is not a causal process; they change together.

Another ontological issue of relevance to a philosophy of evolution is that of levels, or hierarchies. When questioned in interviews for this study, Rogers specifically rejected this concept. However, in her early book, her position appears quite different, more analogous to Teilhard's view. Nearly all evolutionary philosophers believe that man is a unique species, characterized by such qualities as symbolic language, written communication, self-awareness, technological competence, and culture. Even Monod, who has tried to reduce the differences between man and other species to the minimum, is unable to deny the distinctive attributes of man. He resorts to Cartesian dualism, but this is not the only way of describing the uniqueness of man that is available to the philosopher. Teilhard is able to establish the qualitative difference between man and the rest of natue without separating him from the continuity of the universe becoming.

Sellars, Jantsch, and other evolutionary philosophers have described how self-organizing, negentropic systems can reach critical transition points, where sudden and innovative changes occur in the system as a whole. Hierarchies need not impute a greater value to those phases that are further developed in the qualities being descirbed. Rogers, when questioned as to how qualities such as reason and self-awareness have emerged in the course of evolution, said that they are manifestations of pattern (PI, 1). She does not address the reasons why or how pattern can change and manifest new qualities of consciousness. It is likely, however, that this explanation would lie in the integral man/environment process.

The concept of evolution, according to most philosophers, implies an underlying continuity of substance in the process of change. In Monod's view of evolution, this continuity is provided by the self-replication of DNA from one generation to another. In this way, theoretically, all life may have originated from a single DNA molecule. The problems with the continuity of substance—of conscious energy—in Teilhard's worldview have been discussed. Similiar problems occur in Rogers's model. Both Rogers and Teilhard believe that their respective evolutes continue existing after the death of their corresponding physical structure. The difficulty lies in accounting for the appearance of seemingly new evolutes from birth. Where does this apparently new human energy field come from? What is the source of its unique pattern?

Finally, in examining Rogers's ontological implications, the question of what kind of evidence is accepted as legitimate should be addressed. Monod accepts only the objective aspects of existence; he considers no nonmaterial factors or explanations incorporating mental qualities valid. Teilhard accepts both objective and subjective experience as valid, indeed as necesary, data for his synthetic view. Rogers also accepts both objective and subjective data, but seemingly with some limitations. She holds certain kinds of objective data or information irrelevant to a four-dimensional reality. "Empirical evidence . . . . commonly understood to be acquired through 'five-sense perceptible things' . . . . does not reflect the integral nature of human and environmental fields that are manifested in pattern and wave phenomena."[7] On the other hand, Rogers also hesitates to draw upon value-laden or subjective interpretations of the evolutionary process regarding purpose, meaning, first principles, or final causes (PI, 1).

In conclusion, Rogers bases her view of the human energy field in large part on the insights of modern physics, as well as on a philosophy of holism. She expressly rejects reductionism and Cartesian dualism. Harris describes the ontological implications of contemporary physics as follows:

> Matter . . . . has been resolved away into waves and the waves into mathematical formulae . . . . The reality which the physicist investigates has turned out to be of the same essential nature as the activity of thought in which subject and object are one.[8]

Rogers posits an energy manifesting consciousness holistically, nondualistically, and noncausally. This ontology appears to be consistent with Teilhard's ontology of centers of conscious energy.

TELEOLOGICAL IMPLICATIONS OF ROGERS'S MODEL

The implications of Rogers's view of the direction of evolution are related to the teleologial issues of purpose, meaning, value, and causation. Directionality does not necessarily imply purpose or aim, although this can be one of its meanings. One question arising in relation to Rogers's system is, Can there be any direction in a nonlinear, nonspatial, nontemporal realm?

Directionality need not imply linearity; therefore, one can speak to direction as a tendency or trend in a course of events or changes. Because of its linear implications, Rogers avoids use of the term "development." "Process" expresses the same meaning, and Whitehead uses it to avoid linearity:

> There is a prevalent misconception that "becoming" involves the notion of a unique seriality for its advance into novelty. This is the classic notion of "time," which philosophy took over from common sense . . . . Recently physical science has abandoned this notion. Accordingly we should now purge cosmology of a point of view which it ought never to have adoped as an ultimate metaphysical principle.[9]

Rogers also refers to the "life process," which expresses the concept of directional change in a four-dimensional domain.

The only direction Rogers specifies for evolution in her later writings is toward increasing diversity and higher-wave-frequency patterning of the energy field. A synonym for diversity is variety. Rogers states that she is describing the evolutionary trends of the individual human being, but "diversity" is a comparative, or relational term denoting the "condition of being different or having difference."[10] Diversity within oneself would become, then, heterogeneity. Increasing heterogeneity implies an increase in complexity and differentiation. Rogers's delineation of diversity as the direction of evolution must, then, encompass all the terms she prefers to avoid. She, herself, does not deny that these qualities are also increasing in evolution. Therefore, for the purposes of this study, the direction of evolution in Rogers's model will be taken as being toward increasing complexity, heterogeneity, differentiation, and diversity.

Rogers, Teilhard, Whitehear, and Monod are in basic agreement that evolution shows a trend toward increasing complexity. Their disagreement lies in the reasons and meaning they impute to this trend. Teilhard views the increasing complexity as an external or visible manifestation of the increasing personalization of the evolutes. Monod regards the increasing personalization of the evolutes. Monod regards the increasing complexity of the teleonomic apparatus as serving the purpose of reproductive invariance. Whitehead sees it as being impelled by the drive for novelty and intensity of feeling, which is somewhat analogous to personalization. It appears that Rogers's conception of increasing diversity and uniqueness of patterning can be deepened by Teilhard's and Whitehead's descriptions of personalization and subjective intensity. Differentiation and diversity generate more personalized and subjectively distinctive evolutes. This may be what Rogers is implying when she describes evolution as continuously innovative, spontaneous, and creative:

> The creativity of life is a continually evolving phenomenon. Evidence of this creativity finds further expression in the changing dimensions of man's sentience and thought. They are integral to the life process itself. In the process of inter-

action between man and environment, man's self-knowledge and knowledge of his world emerge. (*TBN*, p. 72)

Teilhard's personalization occurs through centration and union, according to the law that "union differentiates." Personalization is creative differentiation. This formulation seems to capture what Rogers is expressing by the concept of increasing diversity. For Teilhard, however, diversity is only the mean by which the primary movement of convergence is attained; "convergence is effected only by means of divergencies that allow life to try everything" (*AE*, p. 124). This view of a converging universe is completely absent from Rogers's model. In this regard, her view is more Bergsonian, describing an endlessly divergent creative process.

In the Teilhardian philosophy, as "the grain of consciousness is personalized, it becomes released from its material support in the phylum" (*AE*, p. 122). One is reminded here of Rogers's correlates of patterning, in which evolution proceeds from materiality to ethereality, pragmatic to visionary, slower field motion to faster. Higer-frequency-wave patterning, apparently, involves a transcendence of human awareness beyond the more dense, slower-wave-patterning of matter, into more subtle, extensive rapid-wave-patterning:

> There are persons whose knowledge of the world is augmented by information gained through other than the five senses. Probably this has been true of visionaries of centuries past as well as now. Today, however, it seems likely that a much larger number of people possess some powers of extrasensory perception. (*TBN*, p. 72)

Not only enhanced perceptive abilities, but a timeless, transcendent awareness "beyond waking" is one of Rogers's postulated correlates of evolution. Cowling studies mystical experience within the Rogerian framework, defining it as "a manifestation of human field patterning as experiential phenomena."[11] Mystical experience was shown by Cowling to be more diverse and associated with higher-frequency-wave patterning. In this regard, it is relevant that ancient Indian yogas are based on the phenomenon of *kundalini*, a nonphysical energy structure in the human being that consists of a hierarchy of vibrating centers, in which the more rapidly vibrating (higher-frequency) centers are associated with a transcendent, subtle, or mystical awareness.[12] In their view of man's evolving into a transcendent of cosmic consciousness, Teilhard and Rogers stand in sharp contrast to Monod. The materialist philosopher is bound to the domain of the five senses and to objective knowledge, which denies any other mode of gaining understanding of the world.

An interesting and related point can be made here, of the similarity between Rogers's four-dimensional reality and the reality experienced in mystical consciousness. Four-dimensional refers, by definition, to a nonlinear, nonspatial, nontemporal domain; furthermore, man and environment in reality are integral, with no boundaries between them. This is the same view of reality revealed in mystical states of awareness. The implications for man's evolution in Rogers's system are, then, that man is becoming increasingly aware of his own true nature and of the nature of the universe. Objective knowledge is not the ultimate way of knowing and does not reveal the essential nature of reality.

Rogers's view of space, time, and three-dimensionality as abstractions of the human mind is not found in the philosphies of Monod or Teilhard who accept space and time as real, and view evolution as a spatiotemporal process. Teilhard holds that there are other realms of existence besides the spatiotemporal; for Rogers, by contrast, all reality is four-dimensional. In this matter, again, her affinity with Bergson is evident, as is her affinity with Eastern philosophies that deny the reality of space and time.[13]

The directionality of evolution must be explained in any evolutionary philosophy; that is, the forces and mechanisms contributing to the progessive changes need to be elucidated. Teleological explanations impute causal efficacy to the purposes, goals, or ends of the process. They do not necessarily imply that a future event of state influences a process taking place in the present. This type of teleogical explanation is rarely seen in modern philosophy. However, Teilhard and Whitehead postulate forces within the evolute and within nature that are purposive or goal-oriented. This is the direct antithesis of Monod's postulate of objectivity, which explains evolution in terms of blind, mechanical process.

Rogers's explanation of directionality falls more in line with those of Teilhard and Whitehead. Her emphasis on the creativity of life and its negentropic repatterning is clearly not in keeping with Monod's conception of chance errors and invariant reproduction. Creativity is a positive force, which is always driving energy fields into self-transcendence, increasing complexity and diversity, and higher-frequency-waves patterns. Whitehead views creativity as the ultimate principle of the universal becoming, whose products have become the phenomenal world. The becoming is a creative (nonserial) advance, in which the many enter into complex unity. Bergson's creative evolution is completely free and indeterminate, with no identifiable trend. Rogers's view of the energy field as negentropic and rhythmically changing precludes complete freedom and indeterminacy. This is why she can speak of probabilistic predictability.

Teilhard and Rogers describe the increasing complexity of their evolutes in very similar language. However Teilhard interprest this as being due to an inner drive toward order that is inherent in the basic energy of the universe. Rogers hesitates to make such an interpretation (PI, 1). However, in a universe devoid of causal processes, a trend of change in any direction is implicitly due to an innate tendency within the evolutes. This is why Monod must find a causal explanation for evolution; without it, he would have to accept innate forces or purpoes. Teilhard's description of the properties of the primordial grain of energy includes the following innate teleological factor:

> a psychic polarization, producing a fundamental tendency to associate with other particles in such a way as to form with them progressively more complex units: the effect of this complexity being (in virtue of a primordial and essential property of cosmic being) to increase simultaneously the degree of immanence in the particle which develops it, and its possibilities of choice (*AE*, p. 133)

Teilhard also speaks of a "self-arranging universe . . . . a drift of the stuff of the cosmos towards states that are continually more complicated physically and more interiorized psychically" (*AE*, p 207). This view is anticpatory of the current paradigm of a self-organizing universe as proposed by Jantsch and others. Rogers's description of the negentropic, rhythmical repatterning and self-transcendence of the human energy field is in a similar train of thought, and the implications of an innate evolutionary trend such as that proposed by Teilhard, are clear.

In marked contrast, however, to Teilhard's view of evolutionary emergence is Rogers's current denial of any levels, or hierarchical unfolding, in the process. Teilhard describes a "tide of convergent psychic energy which rises both qualitatively and quantitatively from isosphere to isosphere, in step with personalization" (*AE*, p. 120). Regardless of whether one views evolution as hierarchical or continuous, the emergence of seemingly new qualities must be explained. Rogers does not explicitly discuss this matter, but some implications from the principles of helicy and integrality can be drawn. The rhythmicity and integrality of the evolute and its environment hold key to the manner in which new properities are generated. Wave phenomena, or rhythmicities, merge into new wave patterns when they interact with each other. Prigogine's research into dissipative structures provides some insight into the manner in which rhythmically fluctuating nonequilibrium systems can suddenly shift into a more orderly pattern when their oscillations reach a critical level. This a noncausal mechanism of change, which seems consistent with Rogers's conception of energy fields as rhythmic phenomena.

The integrality of field and environment can also be seen as a major force of change. In a recent article discussing Rogers's principle of integrality, Wilson and Fitzpatrick discuss the field/environment interaction as a dialectic process in which the inner contradictions among different aspects of the field, and affected by environmental determiners, provide the driving force of evolution.[13]

For Rogers, Teilhard, and Monod, man has the capacity to participate knowledgeably in the evolutionary process. In this respect he must be acknowledged as different from all other life forms. Rogers's conception of higher-frequency-wave patterning can provide an explanation of how human consciousness is able to repattern wave phenomena. The human mind can be described as a subtler, higher-frequency-wave phenomenon than material phenomena. When high frequencies interact with low frequencies, the high-frequency phenomena have a stronger influence on the repatterning that occurs. Mind, within the Rogerian framework, is a holistic, field phenomenon, a manifestation of pattern, which is vibrating at a higher frequency than most other field phenomena. Thus, man, with his highly developed consciousness, becomes an active participant in his own repatterning.

SUMMARY AND CONCLUSIONS

Table 1 provides a summary of Rogers's positions on the ontological and teleological issues discussed in this chapter. In a very general sense, her metaphysic is more comparable to the philosophy of Teilhard than to that of Monod. The differences, however, are also numerous. There are several points of similarity between Rogers's views and those of Bergson and Whitehead. In this section, the above comparisons will be summarized, and final conclusions about the ontology and teleology of Rogers's model will be drawn. Table 2 provides an overview of the comparisons made in this chapter.

The ontological similarities of Rogers's and Teilhard's views are related to their evolving units of organized energy and to their holism. As has been shown, Rogers's view of the energy field implies that the essential nature of the field is one of subjectivity, or consciousness. Hence, and idealistic ontology is closely related to their holism. Because the evolute is an irreducible whole, mind/body dualism is invalid; therefore the modes of awareness manifested by the evolute must be due to an essential property of its basic stuff. As noted earlier, the holistic views of Rogers and Teilhard are similar in two respects. First, the evolute is nondualistic and must be considered an irreducible synthesis of all its qualities and experiences. Second, the evolute is coextensive with the universe, being one aspect of an ultimate wholeness.

The teleological implications of Rogers's model were derived only by extensive analysis of her principle of helicy; it can be said only that they are suggested, but not necessarily required, by her writings and statements. Currently, Rogers prefers not to make any statements as to first principles or final causes. Because she denies any form of external causality in the evolutionary process, the trend toward negentropic repatterning, self-transcendence, and an increasingly subtle and more extensive awareness must be due to innate properties of energy fields. The creativity of the evolutionary process itself must be inherent in the universal becoming. In both these respects, Rogers and Teilhard stand in sharp contrast to Monod.

Ontologically, Rogers differs from Teilhard in her conception of four-dimensionality, which lead to the integrality, infinity, and relativity of the energy field. The boundaries of the energy field are imaginary, and the

TABLE 1
Summary of Rogers's Ontology and Teleology

Onotology	Teleology
1. Evolute: Pattern	1. Causality: Rejected; innate tendencies
2. World-stuff: Energy fields	
3. Mind/body: Dualism rejected; consciousness a manifestation of pattern	2. Entropy/negentrophy: Universe is negentropic
	3. Continuity/hierarchies: Continuity
4. One/many: Integrality; artifical boundaries	4. Death: Patterning is continuous
5. Space/time: Four-dimensionality	5. Direction: Diversity; negentropy; extension of awareness
6. Objectivity/subjectivity: "Experienced as"; relativity	
7. Creativity/mechanism: Rhythmicity, creativity, probability	6. Freedom/determinism: Rhythmicity; man knowledgeable participates
8. Being/becoming: Change is continuous	7. Meaning, value: judgment deferred
9. Holism/reductionism: Irreducibility	
10 Man/nature: Integrality; man not unique	

field is nontemporal, nonspatial, and nonlinear. Field and environment penetrate each other in mutual process. Evolution itself is not a spatiotemporal process, as it is for Teilhard. Rogers and Teilhard also differ in their approach to man's ontological status. For Rogers, man is a type of energy field manifesting certain characteristic properties. For Teilhard, man represents a new qualitative level in a hierarchy of centration and interiority.

The teleological views of Rogers and Teilhard display major differences. Teilhard envisions a converging universe, whereas Rogers sees a diverging universe. The evolutionary process for Teilhard is driven by causal processes, both efficient and final, in Aristotelian terminology. Rogers denies all causality. Finally, for Teilhard, Omega is the ultimate end and fulfillment of the

TABLE 2
Comparison of Rogers with Modern Evolutionary Philosophers

	Monod	Teilhard	Whitehead	Bergson	Rogers
Ontological Issues					
1. The Evolute	Teleonomic apparatus	Psychic centers	Subjective aim, actual occasions	(Forms?)	Patterns, energy fields
2. World-stuff	Invariant molecules	Conscious energy	Prehensions	E'lan vital	Energy fields
3 Mind/Body	Cartesian dualism	Conscious energy	Physical/mental pole	Monism (e'lan)	Rejects dualism
4. One/many	Pluralism	Pluralistic monadism	Many into one	E'lan vital	Integrality
5. Space/time	Only reality	Part of reality	Part of reality	Product of intellect	Four-dimensionality
6. Objectivity/ subjectivity	Objectivity	Interiority	Subjective aim	Intuition	"Experienced as"; relativity
7. Creativity/ mechanism	Chance and necessity	Spontaneity, freedom	Creativity	Freedom creativity	Rhythmicity
8. Being/ becoming	Being (invariance)	Becoming	Process	Becoming	Continuous change

TABLE 2 (continued)

	Monod	Teilhard	Whitehead	Bergson	Rogers
Ontological Issues					
9. Holism/ reductionism	Reductionism	Holism	Holism	Monism	Holism
10. Man/nature	Cartesian dualism	Focus on man	Coextension	—	Integrality
Teleological Issues					
1. Causation	Mechanism	Teleology, mechanism	Subjective aim	Freedom, indeterminacy	Causality rejected; innate tendencies
2. Entropy/ Negentropy	Entropy	Life is negentropic	Increasing complexity	Elan vital	Negentropy
3. Continuity/ hierarchy	Continuity	Emergence	Continuity	Continuity	Continuity
4. Death	Genes are continuous	Irreversible (man)	—	—	Patterning is continuous
5. Direction	Teleonomic complexity	Personalization (convergence)	Novelty and intensity	None	Diversity; negentropy; extension of awareness
6. Freedom/ determination	Determinism; blind chance	Increasing freedom	Increasing freedom	Complete freedom	Rhythmicity; knowledgeable participation by man
7. Meaning, value	Ethic of knowledge	Universe is moral	Permeate the universe	Freedom; intuition	Defers judgment

process of evolution. Rogers places on bounds or ends on the evolutionary process. Self-transcendence is a continual process of change in field patterning.

Certain of Rogers's metaphysical positions resonate with those of Whitehead and Bergson. Whitehead's process philosophy, the philosophy of organism, contains several elements, that are comparable to Rogers's world-view. Creativitiy is the ultimate principle underlying a nonlinear process of progressive integration and intensity of feeling. The subjective aim of an entity organizes its experiences into a self-fulfilling pattern. With Bergson, Rogers shares an emphasis on the diversity and creativity of evolution, and a rejection of space and time as ontological entities.

In the next chapter, and evaluation of the ontological and teleological positions of Rogers's model, elucidated in this chapter, will be presented. To summarize, Rogers's answers to the two questions posed by Russel at the beginning of this chapter might take the following form:

> The universe does have a unity of plan in its evolutionary direction, although no purpose can necessarily be assigned to this plan. Consciousness is indeed, a permanent part of the universe and promise mankind's continous growth in wisdom.

REFERENCES

1. Bertramd Russell, *The Problems of Philosophy* (London: Oxford University Press, 1912), p.155

2. Harris, *The Foundations of Metaphysics in Science*, Part I.

3. *Webster's Seventh New Collegiate Directionay* (Springfield, MA: Merriam, 1971).

4. "Nursing: A Science of Unitary Man," p. 6.

5. Henri Bergson, *Creative Evolution.*

6. Haris, *Nature, Mind and Modern Science.*

7. Francelyn Reeder, "Philosophical Issues in the Rogerian Science of Unitary Human Beings," *Advances in Nursing Science*, 6 (1984), 17–84.

8. *Nature, Mind and Modern Science*, pp. 383–84.

9. *Process and Reality*, p.52.

10. "The Relationship of Mystical Experience, Differentiation and Creativity in College Students," p. 12.

11. Rammurti S. Mishra, *The Textbook of Yoga Psychology* (London: Lyrebird Press, 1972).

12. S. Radhakrishnan, *History of Philosophy Eastern and Western.*

13. Lorraine M. Wilson and Joyce J. Fitzpatrick, "Dialectic Thinking as a Means of Understanding Systems-in-Development: Relevance to Rogers' Principles," *Advances in Nursing Science*, 6, No. 2 (1984), 24–41.

EVALUATION OF ROGERS'S METAPHYSIC

INTRODUCTION

It has been shown that Rogers's evolutionary model is inconsistent with the underlying materialistic metaphysic exemplified by Monod's *Chance and Necessity*. Although in some ways her ontology and teleology approach those of Teilhard, Rogers herself states that she and Teilhard are coming from different worldviews (PI, 1). It appears that Rogers is approaching a new metaphysic in several of her major themes. In a sense, she must define her own reality, within which her views of evolution can be understood. The postulate of four-dimensionality is certainly an effort to describe the general nature of reality, and the principle of integrality also seems to be a step in this direction. Rogers herself suggests that part of her task is metaphysical when she comments that "older cosmologies do not suffice to explain the nature of man and his becoming" (*TBN*, p. 129).

The evaluation of Rogers's ontology and teleology will be guided by Joachim's discussion of systematic coherence, which seems particularly appropriate for a model whose method and content is holistic in character. For Joachim, the conceivability of any element of a science or philosophical system depends on its systematic coherence in relation to the whole:

Thus "conceivability" means for us *systematic coherence,* and is the determining

characteristic of a "significant whole." . . . . Any element of such a whole shares
in this characteristic to a greater or less degree — i.e. is more or less "conceivable"
— in proportion as the whole, with its determinate inner articulation, shines more
or less clearly through that element; or in proportion as the element, in manifesting
itself, manifests also with more or less clearness and fullness the remaining elements
in their reciprocal adjustment.[1]

Joachim explains that "a 'significant whole' is such that all its constituent
elements reciprocally involve one another . . . in a single concrete meaning"
(p. 213). Therefore, in this chapter we will evaluate the systematic coherence
of Rogers's ontology and teleology, in relation to the single or overall meaning of her metaphysic. The first step in this evaluation will be to identify
this overall meaning. With Rogers's general metaphysical theme established,
we will evaluate the ontology and teleology of her model, as identified in
chapter 5, for their systematic coherence.

THE SIGNIFICANT WHOLE OF ROGERS'S MODEL

The attempt to characterize the overall metaphysical them of Rogers's
model led me back to Rogers's earliest book, *Theoretical Basis of Nursing*.
Here, she provides an extensive background and introduction to the model
which forms the foundation for all of her subsequent revisions of the model.
The recurrent theme of this book is present in Rogers's depiction of the life
process of man as characterized by wholeness, continuity, creative change,
unity with nature, and sentience. Although her basic assumptions and principles
have changed since publication of this work, Rogers has retained these basic
qualities of man's evolutionary becoming. Therefore, this characterization of
the life process will be taken as the significant whole of Rogers's model.

It may be helpful to further explore the synthesis of these five attributes
of the life process, in order to encompass them within a single metaphysical
theme. Continuity, creative change, and man's unity with nature are all integral aspects of the concept of evolution. The wholeness and sentience of
the life process can be contained within the philosophical doctrine of personalism, which will be elaborated below.

Personalism may be defined as "a modern term applied to any philosophy
which considers personality the supreme value and the key to the meaning
of reality."[2] Personality, in this context, means the complex unity of conscious experience; it is a holistic concept, not indicative merely of a mental
phenomenon.[3] Fuller explains the distinguishing characteristics of personalism
in the following way:

What would seem to distinguish personalism from other variants of pluralistic
idealism is . . . the overwhelming importance it attributes to the . . . *personal*

characteristics and activities of the individual centers of consciousness, which, with their experiences, constitute Reality . . . . Reality, then, is essentially and primarily a plurality of *personal experients and experiences.*[4]

Human personality is unique and creative, producing and molding its experience freely and responsibly. Personalism involves a holistic approach to knowledge; personal experience as a whole is the source and the ultimate verifier of hypotheses. Personalistic philosophies posit an interacting and intercommunicating universe, life's evolutionary and orthogenetic development, and its inexhaustible potentialities of growth (Brightman, "Personalism").

Rogers's description of the human energy field and its evolutionary repatterning was shown in chapter 5 to imply a process of personalization. It appears that the emphasis placed in her model on the uniqueness of each human field patten, its creative change in the experiential realm, and the holistic nature of human sentience, can appropriately be characterized as personalistic. Rogers believes that the human being is not a physical body, that change is relative for each individual, and that the sense of self is a field manifestation whose nature is unique to each individual. These views are also strongly suggestive that Rogers's concern is personalistic, that she sees the human being as a complex unity of experience with the potentiality for creative change directed from within. In her earlier book, Rogers supports this suggestion when she comments:

> The resolution of health problems and the setting of goals directed toward achieving a healthy people require a new concept of the unity of man and a recognition of man's capacity to feel and reason. Man possesses major resources within himself for determining direction in the developmental process. (*TBN*, p. 134)

Thus, the meaning, or theme that may be assigned to Rogers's metaphysic is an "evolutionary personalism." The following discussion will focus on whether the ontology and teleology of her evolutionary view are coherent in relation to this significant whole of evolutionary personalism.

EVALUATION OF ROGERS'S ONTOLOGY

In Rogers's worldview, the universe consists of energy fields, identified by unique patterns, which are continually changing, creatively and rhythmically. Energy fields are irreducible and are four-dimensional; that is, they are patterned unities that are nonlinear, nonspatial, and nontemporal. Unlike Leibniz's windowless monads, Rogers's energy fields are integral with the universe, in constant mutual process. Furthermore, energy fields possess innate potentialities for self-transcendence, not all of which may be actualized.

The concept of pattern in Rogers's ontology has been shown to contain rich implications for interpretation as the individuating self-awareness, subjectivity, or personality of each energy field. Without the uniqueness of pattern for each energy field, Rogers's ontology would slide into an impersonal, vacuous reality, a sea of energy fields that could not be related to the intense, personal, subjective sense of self experienced in everyday human life. In discussing the development of a specialized science, Whitehead delineates the final stage as being "the introduction of the notion of pattern. Apart from attention to this concept of pattern, our understanding of Nature is crude in the extreme."[5] In this light, it is not surprising that the concept of pattern in Rogers's model is receiving increasing emphasis. Because of its personalizing effect, this stress of pattern is highly consistent with the theme of evolutionary personalism.

Rogers's reluctance to deal with the concept of consciousness is problematic to her ontology, however. It is appropriate that she reject the use of the term in the narrow sense of a particular mental state, for this is related to only one part, rather than to the whole, of the human field. An idealistic ontology, in which the universe is described as consisting of fields of conscious energy, would provide the systematic coherence presently lacking in this area. The global or holistic sense of the word "consciousness"—as awareness, with its three aspects of cognition, conation, and affection—can be used to express the nature of energy at all levels of existence, thus solving the problems associated with any dualistic descriptions of the evolving energy fields of the universe.

In chapter 5, it was shown that this view of consciousness as an innate property of energy fields is strongly implied in Rogers's conception of pattern. Rather than being a manifestation of pattern, consciousness can be called inherent or identical to pattern, since pattern itself is four-dimensional, nonmaterial, irreducible subjectivity. The description of consciousness as a behavior or manifestation of pattern is vulnerable to misinterpretation as a materialistic stance. This poses an additional threat to the systematic coherence of Rogers's ontology, for the overall meaning of her model is the very antithesis of materialism. An energy field that manifests consciousness holistically, nondualistically, and noncausally can properly be described as a field of conscious energy. This ontology would be consistent with Rogers's strong emphasis on the holism and sentience of the human field, and would provide systematic coherence in relation to the theme of evolutionary personalism.

The integrality of each energy field with the environment is consistent with the concept of man's unity with nature. Rhythmical repatterning and self-transcendence provide creative change. However, integrality and continuous repatterning together pose a potential threat to the continuity and personalism of the evolute. The person, the individual, is held to be the particular concern of Rogers's model; yet with imaginary boundaries and continuous repatterning, the individual seems to be dissolving. Again, it may be that describing the evolute as a field of conscious energy may help to preserve the subjective continuity and integrity of the individual, which is necessary for the theme of evolutionary personalism to be adequately reflected.

A similar problem, and potential inconsistency, occurs on the phylogenetic level, in Rogers's rejection of the existence of hierarchies of levels, in the evolutionary repatterning of the universe. She does not give mankind as a unique species its appropriate due. She deemphasizes the distinctive self-awareness and personalization of human beings. This is not true in Rogers's early book, where she amply acknowledged the qualities that differentiate man from other species. In her later writings, however, Rogers does not distinguish man from other animals.

Rogers's claim of humanism and the theme of evolutionary personalism are weakened without a delineation of those qualities that distinguish man from other patterned energy fields. Most philosophers mention such traits as symbolic language, written communication, abstract thought, self-awareness, advanced technology, and culture as distinguishing, even if not necessarily exclusive, characteristics of the human species. Differences can be acknowledged without imputing superiority or inferiority to any species. Hierarchical discussions need not imply linearity or value judgments. In Whitehead's words, "the distinction between man and animals is in one sense only a difference in degree. But the extent of the degree makes all the difference. The Rubicon has been crossed" (*Modes of Thought*, p. 38).

The concept of emergence was discussed in chapter 5 as being one way of approaching the generation of new qualitative levels in the evolutionary process. Rogers refers to emergence in her later writings, but does not formally discuss the mechanisms of emergence, in terms of critical transitions in complexity and consciousness. A full development of this concept would enhance the coherence of her ontology in relation to the theme of evolutionary personalism. Man's intensifying, deepening, personalizing sentience will be encompassed in its full significance, without denying the continuity of the evolutionary process.

To summarize, Rogers's ontology appears to lack coherence—or potentially so—in relation to the theme of evolutionary personalism in two respects. First, her depiction of consciousness as a manifestation of pattern, rather than as inherent in pattern, is suggestive of a materialistc ontology. Second, she does not adequately acknowledge the individual human being as an enduring subjective entity and the human species as a qualitatively new phase of evolution. Revisions of Rogers's ontology that would promote the model's systematic coherence are that the evolute be described as a field of conscious energy, and that the concept of evolutionary emergence be reestablished.

EVALUATION OF ROGERS'S TELEOLOGY

I found Rogers's teleological view relatively undeveloped, but rich with implications. Although she herself delineates only increasing diversity and higher-frequency wave patterning as being the direction of the evolutionary process, it was shown that in a negentropic universe, the direction of change by definition must be toward increasing complexity, heterogeneity, and differentiation. Increasing integration was found to be another necessary concomitant. Finally, on the basis of the correlates of patterning, with their emphasis on an increasingly subtle and more extensive awareness, the principle of helicy was shown to imply an evolutionary direction toward increasing consciousness and complexity, comparable to the Teilhardian view. All of these tendencies, occurring as they do in a noncausal universe, were implied to innate potentialities within energy fields.

The direction of evolutionary change described above, providing that it acknowledges the increasing awareness of the energy field, is consistent with an evolutionary personalism. As discussed in chapter 5, diversity, differentiation, and integration can be seen as aspects of personalization, a deepening intensity of subjective awareness. Even the cosmic or mystical awareness described by both Rogers and Teilhard has a personalizing, rather than a self-annihilating, potential. Expansion and intensification of subjective awareness can occur simultaneously or complementarily.

Rogers's rejection of causality sets her apart from nearly all evolutionary philosophers. It was shown in chapter 5 that the existence of an evolutionary direction in a noncausal universe implies that there are innate potentialities in the evolutes and in the universe. Otherwise, there would be nothing but chaos—random variation, with no discernible order or trend. Evolution, by definition, implies directional change. Therefore, in order to be coherent in relation to an evolutionary personalism, Rogers would need to clarify the existence of innate evolutionary tendencies in conscious energy. With the ontology suggested above, this should pose no logical problem.

The difficulties involved in conceptualizing death in a universe of evolving conscious energy were outlined in chapter 3. Rogers's view of patterning as continuous is consistent with an evolutionary personalism. Birth, the appearance of seemingly new energy fields, may actually be more problematic an issue than death. Rogers does not address this issue, so no conclusion can be made as to its coherence within her model.

Finally, Rogers's avoidance of assigning any meaning or purpose to the evolutionary process requires consideration. Perhaps more than any other aspect of her teleology, this hesitancy must be held to be a threat to the coherence of the significant whole identified as an evolutionary personalism. Again we turn to Whitehead for an illuminating comment on this issue:

> Our experience is a value-experience. . . . The basis of democracy is the common fact of value-experience, as constituting the essential nature of each

> pulsation of actuality. Everything has some value for itself, for others, and for the whole. This characterizes the meaning of actuality. . . . We have no right to deface the value-experience which is the very essence of the universe. Existence, in its own nature, is the upholding of value-intensity. (*Modes of Thought,* pp. 150–51)

In a universe of a holistic, nondualistic nature, value and fact cannot be separated. The very notion that a direction to change can be identified imputes a value of sorts to the quality that is unfolding—that is, to consciousness. Teilhard recognized this and suggested that a new ethic be based on the valuation of consciousness, its enhancement and development.

Harris also recognizes that a view of an evolving universe must attribute a meaning and value to the developmental processes of nature: "The philosophical theory demanded by the modern outlook [of evoluton] must maintain. . . that the ultimate principle of interpretation is, in consequence, the principle of value."[6] That which is unfolding must be held as the measure against which all valuations are made.

Rogers states that one of nursing's goals is to promote the realization of man's maximum health potential. Within her conceptualization of health, one would expect to be able to identify the values inherent in her model. The following statement points toward these values:

> The creativity of life finds expression in man's expanding awareness of the universe and a growing capacity to know his world through paranormal means. Thought and feeling portray man's humanness and underwrite his search for meaning. . . . The world's problems in health. . . must be seen within the context of the incredible magnificence of man's potentials. (*TBN,* p. 138)

Thus, it can be seen that Rogers has indeed identified a value and meaning to the evolutionary process, despite her unwillingness to formalize this. Man's expanding awareness and his search for meaning constitute his unfolding potentialities, and this must be where the meaning of evolution is to be found. All events and conditions can be judged, then, according to whether they contribute to the deepening of human consciousness and sense of meaning. This value system is fully consistent with the significant whole of Rogers's model, the theme of evolutionary personalism.

In summary, Rogers's teleology, if acknowledged and more fully developed, will prove to be consistent with the overall meaning of her model. Specifically, the existence of innate tendencies toward increasing complexity and consciousness within energy fields, and the values and meaning of evolution implied by Rogers's view of human potentials, would fully reflect the significant whole of evolutionary personalism.

REFERENCES

1. Harold H. Joachim, "Truth as Coherence," in *The Nature of Truth* (Oxford: Clarendon, 1906); rpt. in *Contemporary Philosophic Problems,* ed.

Y. H. Krikorian and A. Edel (New York: Macmillan, 1959), p. 214.

2. *The Dictionary of Philosophy,* ed. Dagobert D. Runes (Bombay: Jaico Publishing House, 1957).

3. Edgar Sheffield Brightman, "Personalism," in *A History of Philosophical Systems,* ed. V. Ferm (New York: The Philosophical Library, 1950), pp. 340-52.

4. B. A. G. Fuller, *A History of Philosophy,* 3 ed., p. 524.

5. Alfred North Whitehead, *Modes of Thought* (1938; rpt. New York: Capricorn Books, G. P. Putnam's Sons, 1958), p. 194.

6. *Nature, Mind and Modern Science,* p. 206.

8

STRENGTHENING THE SCIENCE OF
UNITARY HUMAN BEINGS

In relation to the metaphysical spectrum established in earlier chapters, Rogers appears to be more closely related to the modern evolutionary idealists than to the philosophers of the materialist tradition. The key concept of pattern is suggestive of the innateness of consciousness in the world-substance, in harmony with the ontology of Whitehead and Teilhard. In Rogers's view of the direction, purpose, and meaning of evolution, negentropic repatterning is characterized by an increasingly diverse, subtle, and more extensive experiential awareness—again indicating a teleology similar to that of Whitehead and Teilhard.

Perhaps the most unique aspect of Rogers's metaphysic is her characterization of reality as four-dimensional and her rejection of causality. In this she is more extreme than any of the philosophers discussed in the historical review. One certain reason for this is the influence of relativity theory and quantum theory in Rogers's thought. In her earlier writings, it appears that her conception of four-dimensionality was nearly identical to that of Einstein's:

> The human and environmental fields are postulated to be four-dimensional. When Einstein proposed that the three coordinates of space and the coordinate of time be synthesized to arrive at a new dimension—the fourth—and postulated the theory of relativity the universe took on an entirely new look. Newtonian absolutism was

contradicted. The concept of four-dimensionality postulated a world of neither space nor time.[1]

Currently, however, Rogers is intensively elaborating her view of four-dimensionality, and she states that Einstein may not have been describing the same phenomenon: "I don't think he was talking about the same thing I am. But he was talking about synthesizing, and when you synthesize you transcend, you come up with a new product that is irreducible" (PI, 2). Rogers's recent rejection of space and time, in any sense, is more radical than the Einsteinian space-time matrix. Her depiction of the universe as infinite also seems to be different from the boundless, but finite, totality of modern relativistic cosmology.[2] It is possible, of course, that the infinite to which she refers is the expanding universe of relativity, but this point has not been clarified. The purpose of this diversion into relativity is to substantiate the uniqueness of Rogers's metaphysic. Her infinite, four-dimensional world suggests an ontology of rich potentiality, a world-stuff of uniquely patterned—and conscious—energy fields, integral with the universe, in a process of continuous, creative, rhythmical change.

In the previous chapter, evolutionary personalism was identified as the overall theme of the model of unitary human beings. Evolutionary perssonalism is a subset of the philosophical tradition of evolutionary idealism. Since it is somewhat restrictive to limit our discussion only to personalism, the discussion to follow will expand its focus and refer to the larger worldview of evolutionary idealism as an appropriate philosophical theme for Rogers's model. Evolutionary idealism is defined as the view that the fundamental substance of the universe is consciousness, or conscious energy, which is evolving in the direction of higher, more complex, levels of knowledge, feeling, and will (or power).

Rogers's ontology is potentially incoherent in relation to the humanistic metaphysic of evolutionary idealism in two areas. One of these areas is the critical problem of consciousness, which must be dealt with in any evolutionary philosophy. The depiction of consciousness as a manifestation of human field patterning, rather than as an innate quality of the field itself, is suggestive of a materialistic ontology, and is clearly not what Rogers intends to support. Second, the individual human being as an enduring unit of conscious experience and the human species as a unique phase of evolution are not adequately acknowledged. However, Rogers's model can be reinterpreted so that these threats to its humanistic status are eliminated (see pp. 89–91).

The main weakness of Rogers's teleology seems to be its lack of development and clarification. The model is rich with teleological implications, in its principle of helicy, and in Rogers's view of man's health potentials. The existence of an innate tendency to evolve into increasing complexity and consciousness in energy fields, and the values and meaning implied by man's expanding awareness and his search for wisdom, would provide a fuller systematic coherence to the model if they were incorporated.

It is clear that Rogers's intention is to present to the nursing profession a humanistic outlook on the evolving human being that is also in keeping with the most recent scientific insights into the nature of reality. The metaphysical view of evolutionary idealism was found to be highly suitable for this purpose. Specifically, some factors that could be considered for Rogers's ontology and teleology to be more coherent with an evolutionary idealism are as follows:

1. Description of the basic substance of the universe, the fundamental unit of evolution, as a field of conscious energy, identified by its unifying pattern of subjective awareness.

2. Utilization of the concept of evolutionary emergence so that man's unique attributes can be acknowledged without sacrificing his unity with nature.

3. Delineation of the innate tendency within the energy field toward self-transcendence in the direction of increasing personalization and a more extensive and subtle awareness.

4. Acknowledgment of the value-meaning of the evolutionary process that resides in the evolution of consciousness at all levels of existence.

The above factors require further clarification in order to prevent misinterpretation. In regard to the first point, it should be emphasized that the term "conscious energy" is suggested in order to make the point that the later phases of evolution—mind and human consciousness—can be regarded as purely potential and immanent in the world-stuff, not as fully developed actualities. The immanence of consciousness, as a rudimentary awareness, differential reactivity, or subjectivity, in the primordial energy of physics allows the scientific requirement of the continuity and unity of nature to be supported in all phases of evolution. Even in its most elemental forms, energy organizes itself into patterned units. This self-differentiation is the point at which an equally elemental subjectivity can be identified.

The concept of evolutionary emergence to be considered for incorporation into Rogers's model is not the notion suggested by the early emergent evolutionists, in which completely new and unpredictable qualities are introduced in the various phases of the world-process. Rather, the novelty that emerges is attributable to the repatterning of the energy field, which is continuous and rhythmical. This is how Rogers can speak of probabilistic correlates of patterning. In regard to man, then, it cannot be said that he is a new or separate phenomenon, but that his consciousness has reached a new level of operation because of the extreme complexity and integration of his patterning.

The third factor is based on the overwhelming scientific evidence of an evolutionary nisus, present in the very matrix of physical reality, to the formation of increasingly complex forms—"some persistent tendency towards self-enfoldment, self-differentiation, and self-elaboration."[3] This self-differentiation is personalization in Teilhard's terms, diversity in Rogers's. The increasing subtlety and extension of awareness is an integral aspect of this personalization.

Finally, the fourth factor is based on the logic implicit in the concept of evolution, and on Rogers's own discussion of man's evolutionary potential, which resides in his expanding awareness. Harris provides a cogent explanation of the evolutionary logic that allows us to identify the unfoldment of consciousness as the value-meaning of evolution:

> The entire sequence of intertwining processes and changing physical patterns is an organized unity, in which the momentary pattern is continually modified in the direction of greater integrity and completeness. In such a process it is, as always, the organizing principle that dominates and directs, and accordingly the whole is *generated* throughout the process. The course of the process is subject to and each successive phase subserves the increase of complexification and integration. Consequently, the dynamic totality, which at any stage the organism is, issues as a development in which the earlier generates the later and is related to it as means to end. Nevertheless, the means-end relationship between successive phases gives the process its typically teleological appearance and is the reason why the end-state has been emphasized in such teleological movements. It is, however, not its coming last that makes any phase the fulfillment of the process, but its being the most complete and most fully integrated form of the system.[4]

One crucial point must be made: in no way was it intended that human consciousness be considered the final, or ultimate, phase of evolution. This would be completely antithetical to Rogers's open-ended view. However, it does appear that the continuous evolution of consciousness is the locus of value-meaning in her evolutionary vision.

The model of unitary human beings contains profound metaphysical implications and humanistic potentialities unparalleled by any other conceptual model for nursing. The derivation of Rogers's concepts from modern physics may be its greatest strength—and, potentially, its greatest weakness. Certainly, Rogers does not mean to suggest that man is reducible to the laws of physics. The possibility of her model's being interpreted in this way can be avoided if its idealistic implications are acknowledged more fully and incorporated into a metaphysic of evolutionary idealism.

As Rogers's model currently stands, because of its numerous ambiguities and undeveloped ideas, such misinterpretations are possible. Many terms—such as "four-dimensional" and "nontemporal"—are not adequately defined and, being laden with several possible philosophical interpretations, create confusion among students of the model. This study has interpreted the overall meaning of Rogers's outlook as personalistic. However, because of the model's lack of philosophical clarity and consistency, undoubtedly several other interpretations could also be justified. This must be considered a weakness of the model.

The strengths of the model lie in its creativity and fertility as a generator of new approaches to nursing theory, and also in its potential impact on nursing practice. A philosophy for nursing in which the nurse's concern is not only for the physical condition of the client, but also for the client's state of consciousness—for example, the meaning an illness has for the person, and the effect it has on his experience of life and the world—can provide a truly humanistic approach to nursing care. Because of these strengths of the model, it is particulary urgent that attempts be made to clarify and strengthen the model's philosophical base. This study has been one effort to contribute to this task.

REFERENCES

1. "Nursing: A Science of Unitary Man," p. 4 of article.

2. Harris, *The Foundations of Metaphysics in Science,* pp. 64–89.

3. *The Foundations of Metaphysics in Science,* p. 155.

4. *The Foundations of Metaphysics in Science,* p. 267.

IMPLICATIONS FOR THE METAPARADIGM
OF NURSING

Our focus will now turn from Rogers's to other contemporary nursing theories, for in order to justify evolutionary idealism as an appropriate metaparadigm for nursing, we must demonstrate its compatibility with the predominant approach taken by the majority of theories. First, to summarize, the ontological stance of evolutionary idealism is that the fundamental substance of the universe is conscious energy. Post-Darwinian idealists, such as Bergson, Whitehead, and Teilhard, describe conscious energy as being in a process of continual evolution. They characterize human beings by a particular order or level of consciousness that supports their uniqueness, but does not deny their unity with the rest of the universe. They see evolution not as an *exclusively* random, blind selection, but as a process with a clear direction—the unfoldment of greater knowledge-feeling-power.

The worldview of evolutionary idealism has been reflected to varying degrees in a number of nursing theories besides Rogers's. It is most clearly expressed in Newman's theory of health as expanding consciousness. She describes the individual as a "unique pattern of consciousness within a field of absolute consciousness."[1] Newman views disease as an aspect of a "much larger whole that is evolving to a higher order."[2] The evolving, expanding consciousness of the individual develops into levels beyond space-time

101

awareness, which are characterized by love—an extensive and intensive interaction with the universe.

Newman explicitly states her assumption that consciousness resides in all matter. Her definition of consciousness and its connection with space, time, and movement presents philosophical problems that may be resolved by turning to the rigorous thinkers of the evolutionary idealist tradition. This is a task beyond the scope of this chapter. What is important to emphasize here is that Newman's model is highly compatible with the idealist metaphysic and can readily draw support and clarification from it.

Watson's theory of human care is similarly based on an evolutionary perspective of human consciousness. She acknowledges a particular philosophical debt to Whitehead in the development of some key concepts, and also draws upon Teilhard's view of the spiritual evolution of human beings. Watson focuses on the spiritual consciousness of the person as the dimension in need of development through a transpersonal caring relationship between nurse and patient. Care and love make up the basic energy of the universe. The nurse's role is to help a person "gain more self-knowledge, self-control, and readiness for self-healing."[3] Watson appears to view body, mind, and soul as distinct dimensions of a person, implying a holism of parts rather than a strict monism. As is true of all nursing theories, the theory of human care requires greater philosophical clarity and rigor, which again may be facilitated by drawing upon some key concepts of evolutionary idealism.

Consciousness and evolution likewise play central roles in Parse's theory of man-living-health. Parse identifies Rogers's science of unitary human beings and existentialism as her conceptual roots. She describes man as an open being, negentropically unfolding, who freely chooses among options. Health is the unique becoming cocreated by each individual. The evolution of man is toward increasing complexity and diversity. Valuing, imaging, enabling, powering, and transcending are key concepts that can be directly related to a fundamental ontology of consciousness.

Although it is not as readily apparent, Orem's self-care theory of nursing expresses a vew of human beings and health that also finds philosophical support from evolutionary idealism. Orem identifies several points of distinction between human beings and other living things: self-awareness, reflection, symbolization of experience, and symbolic thought. Clearly, the unique order of human consciousness is being addressed in these points. She rejects a dualistic view of mind and body, describing the person as "a unity that can be viewed as functioning biologically, symbolically, and socially."[4] Human development proceeds toward higher and higher levels of integration of physical, psychic, and intellectual characteristics. Self-care, in its fullest sense, requires a highly developed consciousness (knowledge-feeling-power). Thus, evolutionary idealism may provide a useful philosophical foundation for this model.

The above analysis of the appropriateness of evolutionary idealism as a philosophical foundation for the majority of nursing theories brings this book full circle—back to its stated goal of clarifying and strengthening the metaphysical foundations of nursing science. In chapter 1, the necessity of developing a philosophical foundation for nursing's metaparadigm was defended. A *unified* worldview was identified as a desirable goal for maintaining the status of an academic discipline. Through the intensive analysis of the model of unitary human beings and its relationship to the spectrum of evolutionary philosophy, some important philosophical issues have been clarified and certain metaphysical positions have been identified as being particularly appropriate for the holistic, evolutionary, and humanistic approach of Rogerian science. These same metaphysical stances will now be explored for their relevance in explicating a metaparadigm for nursing.

There has occured in recent years an implicit—and often explicit—rejection of materialism as being a worldview inappropriate for nursing. This has most frequently taken the form of a rejection of quantitative, reductionistic, and dualistic approaches to nursing research. Nursing theorists emphasize the concepts of holism, development, and humanism, all of which are directly supported by the philosophy of evolutionary idealism. This book has attempted to provide extensive philosophical argumentation against materialism, and has offered an alternative metaphysical foundation for the discipline of nursing. Further philosophical discussion of the ideas presented here should lead to a solid and rigorous metaparadigm. Nurse philosophers—current and future—are invited to continue intensive exploration of the issues raised in this work.

REFERENCES

1. Margaret A. Newman, *Health as Expanding Consciousness* (St. Louis: C. V. Mosby, 1986), p. 20.

2. *Health as Expanding Consciousness,* p. 22

3. Jean Watson, *Nursing: Human Science and Human Care* (Norwalk, CT: Appleton-Century-Crofts, 1985), p. 35.

4. Dorothea E. Orem, *Nursing: Concepts of Practice,* 2 ed. (New York: McGraw-Hill, 1980), p. 120.

BIBLIOGRAPHY

Philosophy

Anthony, G. F. Penn, "Whither Evolution? Some Questions to Teilhard de Chardin." *International Philosophical Quarterly,* No. 15 (March, 1975), pp. 71–82.

Aristotle. *Aristotle: Selected Works,* Trans. and ed. R. P. Hardie and R. K. Gaye. New York: Random House, 1941.

_____. *Metaphysics.* Trans. R. Hope. New York: Columbia Univ. Press, 1952.

Armour, L. *The Concept of Truth.* Assen: Van Gorcum and Co., 1969.

Aurobindo, S. *The Life Divine.* 3rd ed. New York: India Library Society, 1965.

Ayer, A. J. *Language, Truth and Logic.* 1936; rpt. New York: Dover, 1946.

Barbour, I. G. *Issues in Science and Religion.* New York: Harper & Row, 1966.

Bergson, H. *Creative Evolution.* Trans. A. Mitchell. 1907; rpt. New York: Random House, 1944.

Bhattacharya, A. C. *Sri Aurobindo and Bergson: A Synthetic Study.* Varanasi, India: Jagabhandu Prakashan, 1972.

Birx, J. K. *Pierre Teilhard de Chardin's Philosophy of Evolution.* Springfield, MA: Charles C. Thomas, 1972.

Bohm, D. *Wholeness and the Implicate Order.* London: Routledge & Kegan Paul, 1980.

Bonifazi, C. *The Soul of the World: An Account of the Inwardness of Things.* Washington, DC: University Press of America, 1978.

105

Brightman, E. S. "Personalism." In *A History of Philosophical Systems.* Ed. V. Ferm. New York: The Philosophical Library, 1950.

Burnett, J. *Early Greek Philosophy.* 4th ed. London: Adam & Charles Black, 1930.

Canfield, J. V., ed. *Purpose in Nature.* Englewood Cliffs, NJ: Prentice-Hall, 1966.

Carse, J. C. *Death and Existence: A Conceptual History of Human Mortality.* New York: Wiley, 1980.

Chaucard, P. *Man and Cosmos: Scientific Phenomenology in Teilhard de Chardin.* New York: Herder and Herder, 1965.

Darwin, C. *Origin of Species.* 1864; rpt. New York: New American Library, 1958.

Delaney, C. F. *Mind and Nature: A Study of the Naturalistic Philosophy of Cohen, Woodbridge and Sellars.* Notre Dame: Univ. of Notre Dame Press, 1969.

Descartes, René. *Meditations on First Philosophy.* Trans. E. S. Haldane and G. R. T. Ross, from 2nd Latin ed. (1642). In *The Philosophical Works of Descartes.* 1911; rpt. Cambridge: Cambridge Univ. Press, 1972. Vol. I.

Dewey, J. *Experience and Nature.* 2nd ed. 1929; rpt. New York: Dover, 1958.

Dobzhansky, T. "Teilhard de Chardin and the Orientation of Evolution." *Zygon,* 3 (1968), 242–58.

Doud, R. E. "Wholeness as Phenomenon in Teilhard de Chardin and Merleau-Ponty," *Philosophy Today,* 24 (1980), 90–103.

Fabel, A. *Cosmic Genesis: Teilhard de Chardin and the Emerging Scientific Paradigm.* Teilhard Studies Number 5. Chambersburg, PA: Anima, 1981.

Falckenbert, R. *History of Modern Philosophy.* 3rd ed. Trans. A. C. Armstrong. Calcutta: Progressive Publishers, 1953.

Fuller, B. A. G. *A History of Philosophy.* 3rd ed. Rev. by S. M. McMurrin. New York: Henry Hold, 1955.

Gentner, D. R. "The Scientific Basis of Some Concepts of Pierre Teilhard de Chardin." *Zygon,* 3 (1968), 432–44.

Glowienka, E. "Notes on Consciousness in Matter." *New Scholasticism,* 43 (1969), 602–13.

Goodman, L. E., and M. J. Goodman, "Creation and Evolution: Another Round in an Ancient Struggle." *Zygon,* 18 (1983), 3–43.

Gould, S. J., and N. Eldredge, "Punctuated Equilibria: The Tempo and Mode of Evolution Reconsidered." *Paleobiology,* 3 (1977), 115–51.

Happold, F. C. *Mysticism.* 2nd ed. London: Penguin, 1967.

Harris, E. E. *The Foundations of Metaphysics in Science.* 1965; rpt. Lanham, MD: University Press of America, 1983.

_____. *Nature, Mind and Modern Science*. London: George Allen & Unwin, 1954.

Hastings, J., ed. *Encyclopedia of Religion and Ethics*. New York: Scribner, 1961.

Hoffding, H. *A History of Modern Philosophy*. Trans. B. E. Meyer. 2 vols. 1895; rpt. New York: Dover, 1955.

Hull, D. *Philosophy of Biological Science*. Foundations of Philosophy Series. Englewood Cliffs, NJ: Prentice-Hall, 1974.

Huxley, J. *Evolution in Action*. 1953; rpt. New York: Harper, 1966.

Jantsch, E., ed. *The Evolutionary Vision*. AAAS Selected Symposia Series, 61. Boulder, CO: Westview, 1981.

Jensen, U. J. and R. Harre, eds. *The Philosophy of Evolution*. New York: St. Martin's, 1981.

Joachim, H. H. "Truth as Coherence." In *The Nature of Truth*. Oxford: Clalrendon, 1906. Rpt. in *Contemporary Philosophic Problems*. Ed. Y. H. Krikorian and A. Edel. New York: Macmillan, 1959.

Joad, C. E. M. *Guide to Philosophy*. New York: Dover, 1936.

King, U. *Towards a New Mysticism: Teilhard de Chardin and Eastern Religions*. London: Collins, 1980.

Koestler, A. and J. R. Smythies, eds. *Beyond Reductionism*. New York: Macmillan, 1969.

Laszlo, E. *The Systems View of the World*. New York: Braziller, 1972.

Leibniz, G. W. *Selections*. Ed. P. Wiener. New York: Scribner, 1951.

Lewis, J. L., ed. *Beyond Chance and Necessity: A Critical Inquiry into Professor Jacques Monod's Chance and Necessity*. Atlantic Highlands, NJ: Humanities Press, 1974.

Melsen, A. van. *Evolution and Philosophy*. Pittsburgh: Dusquesne Univ. Press, 1965.

Miles, J. A. "Jacques Monod and the Cure of Souls." *Zygon,* 9 (1974), 22–43.

Mishra, R. S. *The Textbook of Yoga Psychology*. London: Lyrebird, 1972.

Monod, J. *Chance and Necessity*. Trans. A. Wainhouse. New York: Knopf, 1971.

Nagel, E. *The Structure of Science*. New York: Harcourt, Brace & World, 1961.

Needham, J. *Order and Life*. 1936; rpt. Cambridge: MIT Press, 1968.

O'Conner, J. ed., *Modern Materialism: Readings on Mind-Body Identity*. New York: Harcourt, Brace & World, 1969.

O'Manique, J. *Energy in Evolution*. New York: Humanities Press, 1969.

Polanyi, M. *The Study of Man*. Chicago: Univ. of Chicago Press, 1959.

Potter, V. R. "Teilhard de Chardin and the Concept of Purpose." *Zygon,* 3 (1968), 367–76.

Price, H. H. "Clarity Is Not Enough." *Proceedings of the Aristotelian Society,* Supp. Vol. XIX (1945). Rpt. in *Contemporary Philosophic Problems*. Ed. Y. H. Krikorian and A. Edel. New York: Macmillan, 1959.

Prigogine, I. *From Being to Becoming*. San Francisco: Freeman, 1980.

Quintelier, G. "Ideal Objectivity, Modern Biology and Technical Innovation." *Man and World,* 14 (1981), 369–85.

Radhakrishnan, S., ed. *History of Philosophy Eastern and Western*. London: George Allen & Unwin, 1952.

Ramanand, S. *Evolutionary Spiritualism*. Bisalpur, India: Sadhana Karyalaya, 1956.

Randall, J. H. and J. Buchler. *Philosophy: An Introduction*. New York: Barnes & Noble, 1942.

Rensch, B. *Biophilosophy*. Trans. C. A. M. Sym. New York: Columbia Univ. Press, 1971.

Riggan, G. "Testing the Teilhardian Foundations." *Zygon,* 3 (1968), 259–90.

Runes, D. D. *The Dictionary of Philosophy*. Bombay: Jaico, 1957.

Russell, B. *A History of Western Philosophy*. New York: Simon & Schuster, 1945.

————. *Mysticism and Logic*. 1917; rpt. Garden City, NY: Doubleday Anchor Books, 1964.

————. *The Problems of Philosophy*. London: Oxford Univ. Press, 1912.

Sellars, R. W., ed. *Philosophy for the Future: The Quest of Modern Materialism*. New York: Macmillan, 1949.

Shapiro, R. "The Origin of Life." Manuscript submitted for publication, 1983.

Spinoza, B. de. *Ethics*. Ed. J. Gutmann. New York: Hafner, 1949.

Stace, W. T. *The Teachings of the Mystics*. New York: Mentor Books, New American Library, 1960.

————. *A Critical History of Greek Philosophy*. London: Macmillan, 1920.

Stiernotte, A.P. "An Interpretation of Teilhard as Reflected in Recent Literature." *Zygon,* 3 (1968), 377–425.

Taylor, R. *Metaphysics*. Foundations of Philosophy Series. Englewood Cliffs, NJ: Prentice-Hall, 1974.

Teilhard de Chardin, Pierre. *Activation of Energy.* Trans. R. Hague. London: Collins, 1970.

_____. *The Future of Man.* Trans. N. Denny. New York: Harper & Row, 1964.

_____. *Human Energy.* Trans. R. Hague. New York: Harcourt Brace Jovanovich, 1969.

_____. *The Phenomenon of Man.* Trans. B. Wall. New York: Harper, 1965.

Turley, P. T. *Peirce's Cosmology.* New York: Philosophical Library, 1977.

Underhill, E. *Mysticism.* 12th ed. 1910; rpt. Cleveland: Meridian Books, World, 1970.

Warner, R. *The Greek Philosophers.* New York: New American Library, 1958.

Webster's Seventh New Collegiate Dictionary. Springfield, MA: Merriam, 1971.

Whitehead, A. N. *Modes of Thought.* 1938; rpt. New York: Capricorn Books, Macmillan, 1958.

_____. *Process and Reality.* 1929; rpt. New York: Harper, 1960.

Whittaker, J. *The Neo-Platonists.* Cambridge Univ. Press, 1901.

Widgery, A. G. "Classical German Idealism, The Philosophy of Schopenhauer and Neo-Kantianism." In *A History of Philosophical Systems.* Ed. V. Ferm. New York: The Philosophical Library, 1950.

Nursing

Carper, B. A. "Fundamental Patterns of Knowing in Nursing." *Advances in Nursing Science,* 1, No. 1 (1978), 13–24.

Chance, K. S. "Nursing Models: A Requisite for Professional Accountability." *Advances in Nursing Science,* 3, No. 1 (1980), 57–65.

Chinn, P. L., and Maeona K. Jacobs, "A Model for Theory Development in Nursing." *Advances in Nursing Science,* 3 No. 1 (1980), 1–12.

Cowling, R. "The Relationship of Mystical Experience, Differentiation and Creativity in College Students." Diss. New York University, 1982.

Crawford, G., S. K. Dufault, and E. Rudy. "Evolving Issues in Theory Development." *Nursing Outlook,* 27 (1979), 346–51.

Donaldson, S. K. and D. M. Crowley. "The Discipline of Nursing." *Nursing Outlook,* 26 (1978), 113–20.

Downs, F., and J. Fleming. *Issues in Nursing Research.* New York: Appleton-Century-Crofts, 1979.

Duffey, M., and A. Muhlenkamp. "A Framework for Theory Analysis." *Nursing Outlook,* 22 (1974), 570–74.

Ellis, R. "Characteristics of Significant Theories." *Nursing Research,* 17 (1968), 217–23.

_____. "Conceptual Issues in Nursing." *Nursing Outlook,* 30 (1982), 406–10.

Fawcett, J. "The Relationship Between Theory and Research: A Double Helix." *Advances in Nursing Science,* 1, No. 1 (1978), 49–62.

_____. *Analysis and Evaluation of Conceptual Models of Nursing.* Philadelphia: F. A. Davis, 1984.

Feldman, H. R. "Nursing Research in the 1980s: Issues and Implications." *Advances in Nursing Science,* 3, No. 1 (1980), 85–92.

_____. "A Science of Nursing: To Be or Not to Be?" *Image,* 13 (1980), 63–66.

Flaskerud, J. H., and E. J. Halloran. "Areas of Agreement in Nursing Theory Development." *Advances in Nursing Science,* 3, No. 1 (1980), 1–8.

Gortner, S. R. "Nursing Research: Out of the Past and Into the Future." *Nursing Research,* 29 (1980), 204–207.

_____. "Nursing Science in Transition." *Nursing Research,* 29 (1980), 180–83.

Griffin, A. P. "Philosophy and Nursing." *Journal of Advanced Nursing,* 5 (1980), 261–72.

Hardy, M., ed. *Theoretical Foundations for Nursing.* New York: MSS Information Corp., 1973.

Jacobson, S. F. "A Semantic Differential for External Comparison of Conceptual Nursing Models." *Advances in Nursing Science,* 6, No. 2 (1984), 58–70.

Jacox, A. "Theory Construction in Nursing." *Nursing Research,* 23 (1974), 4–13.

Johnson, D. E. "The Behavioral System Model for Nursing." In *Conceptual Models for Nursing Practice,* 2nd ed. Ed. J. Riehl and C. Roy. New York: Appleton-Century-Crofts, 1980.

_____. "Development of Theory: A Requisite for Nursing as a Primary Health Profession." *Nursing Research,* 23 (1974), 372–77.

King, I. *Toward a Theory for Nursing.* New York: Wiley, 1971.

Leininger, M. M. "Nature, Rationale, and Importance of Qualitative Research Methods in Nursing." In *Qualitative Research Methods in Nursing.* Ed. M. Leininger. Orlando, FL: Grune & Stratton, 1985.

Manchester, P. "Analytic Philosophy and Foundational Inquiry: The Method." In *Nursing Research: A Qualitative Perspective.* Ed. P. Munhall and C. Oiler. Norwalk, CT: Appleton-Century-Crofts, 1986.

Meleis, A. I., and K. May. "Nursing Theory and Scholarliness in the Doctoral Program." *Advances in Nursing Science,* 4, No. 2 (1981), 31–45.

Munhall, P. L. "Nursing Philosophy and Nursing Research: In Apposition or Opposition?" *Nursing Research,* 31 (1982), 176–81.

Newman, M. *Theory Development in Nursing.* Philadelphia: F. A. Davis, 1979.

Orem, D. *Nursing Concepts of Practice.* 2nd ed. New York: McGraw-Hill, 1980.

Reeder, F. "Philosophical Issues in the Rogerian Science of Unitary Human Beings." *Advances in Nursing Science,* 6, No. 2 (1984), 14–23.

Rogers, M. E. "Nursing: A Science of Unitary Man." In *Conceptual Models for Nursing Practice.* 2nd ed. Ed. J. Riehl and C. Roy. New York: Appleton-Century-Crofts, 1980

————. "Beyond the Horizon." In *The Nursing Profession: A Time to Speak.* Ed. N. Chaska. New York: McGraw-Hill, 1982.

————. *An Introduction to the Theoretical Basis of Nursing.* Philadelphia: F. A. Davis, 1970.

————. "Nursing Science: A Science of Unitary Human Beings, Glossary." Unpublished paper, 11/22/82.

————. Personal Interview, December 12, 1983.

————. Personal Interview, January 31, 1984.

————. "Science of Unitary Human Beings: A Paradigm for Nursing." In *Family Health: A Theoretical Approach to Nursing Care.* Eds. I. W. Clements and F. B. Roberts. New York: Wiley, 1983.

Roy. C. *Introduction to Nursing: An Adaptation Model.* 2nd ed. Englewood Cliffs, NJ: Prentice-Hall, 1984.

Roy, C., and S. L. Roberts. *Theory Construction in Nursing: An Adaptation Model.* Englewood Cliffs, NJ: Prentice-Hall, 1981.

Schlotfeldt, R. M. "The Need for a Conceptual Framework." In *Nursing Research I.* Ed. P. J. Verhonick. Boston: Little, Brown, 1975.

Schwab, J. "Structure of the Disciplines: Meanings and Significances." In *The Structure of Knowledge and the Curriculum.* Eds. G. W. Ford and L. Pugno. Chicago: Rand McNally, 1964.

Silva, M. "Philosophy, Science, Theory: Interrelationships and Implications for Nursing Research." *Image,* 9 (1977), 59–63.

Stevens, B. *Nursing Theory.* Boston: Little, Brown, 1979.

Watson, J. *Nursing: Human Science and Human Care.* New York: Appleton-Century-Crofts, 1985.

_____. "Nursing's Scientific Quest." *Nursing Outlook,* 29 (1981), 413–16.

Wilson, L., and Joyce Fitzpatrick. "Dialectic Thinking as a Means of Understanding Systems-in-Development: Relevance to Rogers' Principles." *Advances in Nursing Science,* 6, No. 2 (1984), 24–41.

APPENDIX

Transcripts of Interviews with Dr. Rogers

December 12, 1983

BJS: At various times and places, you have described evolution as proceeding toward increasing diversity, differentiation, complexity, and higher-frequency-wave pattern. Do you still believe that all of these are increased in evolution?

MER: I am well aware that they are not [interchangeable] in any kind of specificity. "Diversity," as a single term, says it better, and I think there will be less confusion. Before, I thought, "Well, you know, maybe if one word doesn't catch them, another one will." But, in particular, the term "complexity," I think, people seem to define in many different ways. So, after much thinking, I settled on "diversity."

BJS: Will you be defining "diversity" in a very specific way?

MER: No, I am using it in the general language sense. And, as matter of fact, there will probably be two or three terms, in addition to these, that I will define—"wave frequency" is one that people seem to be having a lot of trouble with, so I may define that one. I think that definitions, if there are too many, end up being jargon. What I would like people to do is to go back to the general language. Because in no way does how I use these terms refer to anything in physics or biology or anything.

One thing that I was interested in: somewhere you said that you had a feeling that maybe mine would fall between Teilhard de Chardin's and Monod's. I would propose that it won't fall between them, because they both derive from different worldviews than the one I believe in, and it

113

will be over here, to the side someplace. It's simply that it isn't a question of hierarchies or anything. It's just that they each had their own view of what they thought things were like.

Those who are committed to Monod's approach—while I think they're all wrong—certainly have a perfect right to do it and, certainly, I think he stated his case very well. So, although I disagree with just about everything he said, I admire his ability to state it.

Now, the wave pattern—it's "patterning" that is the operative word. In those correlates that I gave you, you see, "correlates of patterning." And the definition of "pattern" has been changed, and I'm trying to be very careful that I don't use "pattern" anywhere in the book except when I mean specifically this, because "pattern" has a lot of different meanings in the general language. So I'm just simply using another word if I want something else. So that, in the book, or in talks, or whatever I do, I'm trying to limit the use of this word to only those instances where this is what it means. And then it ties in with this, as well. In other words, it is a word of specificity for this particular science.

BJS: What do you mean when you say it's an operative word?

MER: I mean that it's that which is important, not the "wave frequency." And one of the things that I've been running into more and more is that people want to interpret "wave frequency" like "t" waves or "p" waves or physics or something like that, which of course has no relevance. Wave, itself, is—I haven't decided what to do with it—but it's an abstraction, nobody has ever seen one. And I use it really more—the frequency and wave—as general language to get across the idea of nonrepeating rhythmicities and acceleration. But it's the pattern that is really important. I've tried various definitions, but nothing good has come out yet. But give me time. If I get it before you are done, you shall have it. I would like to have this thing finished and at the publisher's before the end of the year, so it's going to come around—or else!

BJS: It's good to know, because I had always thought of waves—since you spoke of energy and energy fields—somehow I had connected waves with energy—as energy waves.

MER: Well, in a sense they are because, in the abstract sense, they're a manifestation of pattern. And certainly energy is integral to the system. And I know, later on, you raised the question; you got into electromagnetic energy, which you can just cross out of that book. I have defined energy field—what I mean by it—and it's really more a general language definition in which it's the fundamental unit. Field is a unifying concept; energy signifies it is dynamic. Energy fields are infinite, so these are really infinite dynamic unity or some such silly stuff. Does that clarify it?

BJS: Yes. Now, when you say they are infinite, does that mean in terms of their boundaries? Or, there are no boundaries, I know. So that's what infinite refers to, really, infinite in time, as well as in space, but not really spatial or temporal.

MER: There is no space or time in this system. All those are man-made concepts. And even in some of the other sciences—like physics, for example—they keep pointing out that there is no such thing as universal time. We have planet time by atomic clocks, or whoever is measuring what, but they have no relevance as far as the universe goes. It's just something that gets us to a point—some meals on time. Actually, in the literature one can find definitions of energy fields as being infinite. Back in 1969, electromagnetic was a big "in" thing, and so I did what everybody else was doing, because I didn't know any better, either. Well, that's outdated, and a very narrow concept, and so I haven't used it in a good while. So forget I ever said it. The basic framework in that book [Rogers, An Introduction to the Theoretical Basis of Nursing, 1970] was good. And of course there's just so much more data now that supports the direction of this worldview, I think I'm ahead of the game. That's my own bias.

BJS: What are the interrelationships among diversity, differentiation, complexity, and wave pattern?

MER: On this, it isn't that there are interrelationships among these; but the diversity is a manifestation of field pattern. Then I think that, as far as I was able to go, I told you what I mean by that higher-frequency business.

BJS: How do you explain the above-mentioned direction of evolutionary change? Why or how does it occur?

MER: I think one of the things I get into (I don't talk about unidirectionality anymore for a lot of reasons, one being, again, it's confusing and people tend to want a linear, longitudinal sort of thing, which is not what I have in mind), I think one thing I might mention here—I don't deal with first principles or final endings. I don't know what they are, anybody's guess is as good as mine, and there are guesses all over the place. So I wouldn't know. All I'm saying is that, based on present knowledge that I possess—whatever that is—this is the way the world looks to me—like it is—being fully aware that in another 20 years we're going to know a lot of things we don't know now. Things may change. In fact, I'm sure they will change. But it does seem to me, as a unifying paradigm, that this is going to last for a little while. Now, maybe when we get up there and meet those little green men, why, I don't know what we will have. So when I talk about the direction, all I'm really saying is that—and your design seemed to me to pick that up, too—it's in the direction of growing diversity of field pattern.

In that sense, one of the things I've been trying to do and, I don't know, I guess I need an artist, I think there are ways that I could use analogies, or drawings, or whatever, to get across a point; it would help. So when I talk about the human and environmental fields being integral with one another, you see I was caught in my own obsolete thinking when I talked about boundaries; there is no such thing if you are talking about a universe of open systems—and talking about integralness and all this sort of thing. I've been thinking about the possibility of plastic overlays. If you had one that was an infinite environmental field that had some kind of a pattern and then put the overlay on it that was the human field that infinite, with its pattern, they would both be integral. I don't want to say extend to, because that's a spatial term—they simply are integral. The only thing that is different about them is the pattern. And they are in continual mutual process with patterning changing continuously—and these, of course, are four-dimensional, which means that they are—so it doesn't derive from the old spatial or temporal constructs. Also, you'd better not blame Einstein for what I did. But I see them as they're always changing together. They're unique because—there is the arbitrary saying that human beings and their environment are what we are concerned with. I think that you mentioned, somewhere, that this be just one thing. But if one is wanting to study something, one can arbitrarily specify the phenomenon. So that, actually, I have two phenomena that I'm concerned with, human and environmental, and they're always unique, and the human and environmental fields are in concert, if you like, so it's not "if A then B." One doesn't cause the other to change. They change. Now, if you ask me why they change, I don't know. There are a lot of things I don't know. In fact, I suspect I'll die not knowing.

BJS: In a universe of noncausality, how are we able to find a direction in evolution? Is there an innate trend?

MER: All I'm really saying is that, certainly, on the basis of observation and speculation and theorizing, it's going on, and the thing I get into with those building blocks, or postulates—and I'm calling them postulates instead of assumptions—I am saying that I simply postulate energy fields, etc., and they're four. The business of noncausality again isn't a new idea. I'm sure you got that little quote I was handing out in classes—Bertrand Russell. He's so funny. He says things so well—an artist with words. As a matter of fact, causality went out and acausality came in when quantum theory began. But we are dealing with the sacred cows of scientists, and they are going to give it up with great reluctance—even when the evidence is there. But if you have these four-dimensional energy fields—and by definition energy fields are open—and if they are infinite, then one does have a universe that is open.

BJS: Could you elaborate on your view of the phenomena of entropy and negentropy in the universe?

MER: Entropy and negentropy I've used more in the sense of how different people have used them. Certainly in the world of physics it means running down. Entropy derives from a closed-system model of the universe. Negative entropy, I always tend to give von Bertalanffy the credit for it, although there were others who were proposing similar kinds of ideas at about the same time. He left the universe closed, but he said that living systems were open, that they didn't act that way. But, then, he still left them closed at the end, because they eventually had to run down. So he, too, was dealing with a closed-system universe. I think, in a sense, some of that was what Prigogine was doing when he proposed nonrepeating, noncausality, and all of the work he did when he got his Nobel Prize. He was trying to look at what happened with living systems in a closed-system universe, and he proposed that these things could go on. In that he sense he supported [open systems], but didn't go as far, where I propose that the universe is not closed. Now, certainly, there is supporting evidence from various scientists. It's been reported in science journals and *Time* magazine, and they also point out that, when this evidence gets into the general purview, the traditional house of physics is going to fall down like a deck of cards. Because the whole body of knowledge in physics is based on a closed-system model. And so it's going to go. The evidence is creeping up all the time. It's not a new idea, and I think a lot of it. People operate on a very narrow base, so they say, "It looks that way, so it has to be so." So it's no more valid than the people who wanted to burn Galileo at the stake. I think they're going to be sending this causality business. I think that the critical mass is about here. So, I use those terms essentially like this: entropy is a closed-system concept and negative entropy is an open-system concept. Then I give it considerably more scope than von Bertalanffy or the others who went along with this.

BJS: So you would say that the entire universe is negentropic?

MER: Yes. But it's not a middle regions sort of deal, that sometimes people have tried to use as a means of getting around contradictions. I'm just saying that that's it.

BJS: What is the difference between life and nonlife? Man and animals?

MER: I don't think man and animals are any different. I don't know the difference between life and nonlife. And I've used it in a pretty gross sort of way. One of the things that I will be removing from that book, I'm not going to talk about man being at the peak of anything. I don't know whether he is or not; we're pretty conceited. But we are different. And I'm removing all the hierarchical sort of things. I'm concerned with people and their environment. One could study any animal this way if one wanted to arbitrarily say, "This is what I want to look at." Cell physiologists study cells as field units. Certainly, if one looks at what people get into, the micro-micro-microscopic, there comes a point at which they can't tell the difference. So the people who try to catalogue all of these, one year they'll list it under the "life" and the next year under the "nonlife." And then somebody will come along and switch it. I would not want to say that it is a continuum, because here again it gets into linear thinking. I guess I would say that it's a manifestation of pattern; but I don't plan to discuss it, because I don't think it's relevant. Now, in some future day I might want to look at it that way. So I'm talking about human beings, rather than other animals, because man is an animal in the general sense. I think the gap sort of disappeared, at least for scientists, some time ago—20, 30, 40 years ago.

BJS: So, man is not really further along; that's a linear view again. Would man be more diverse than animals? Man as a species?

MER: I don't know. You know, there are other animals who have capacities that we don't have—like hearing sound, and perceiving earthquakes, and flying in the air, and all sorts of things. So what we have is tremendous diversity in the manifestations of life. And I don't think it really matters, certainly not at this moment. I think one of the things, whether one is dealing with it on an everyday basis of looking at the manifestations of the universe, respect for difference becomes increasingly important. And I would say this has not been a characteristic of people, nor is it now very pervasive. Everybody wanted to be the same, and we placed high values, and people wanted to live up to the Joneses, or whatever. In that kind of sense, everybody wanted to be at the top; but being average, in the sense of being normal or alike, has been where the emphasis has been. I would say that I do not value that. Considering that I believe change is accelerating—has already accelerated rapidly—we've had a very short period of time with the bell curve, which is already invalid for describing populations. It's almost as though we went through a brief plateau and now it's gone, like the wind. I think that trying to differentiate between these is all right for somebody that wants to do it, but comparative dissertations between man and other animals and between life and nonlife, I'll leave to somebody else. I think that they try to do it on gross observation, not on any kind of depth thinking; and I think that it's generally been more a mechanistic approach. Now of course, man and other animals, it's been religion and philosophy and most anything anybody wanted to toss into the bucket, and a little fear and conceit and all sorts of things. I think we should value all of them. I don't think one knows people. We ask so many wrong questions, and when people tried to say how man was different from other animals, they didn't get very far. I grew up in eastern Tennessee, where "evolution" was a bad word—the Monkey Trial. In zoology class they weren't allowed to teach evolution. But I learned evolution in comparative anatomy, because the teacher had a leg bone of a horse, and a leg bone of a cow, and of a man, and he said, "I wanted you to notice, they're none of them the same." But they all looked alike to me! My concern is with synthesis, not analysis. I think we wear out the categorizations.

BJS: What do you mean by evolution from the pragmatic to the visionary?

MER: Now on that, from pragmatic to visionary, if you look at those correlates, this "frequency" will be removed, in the sense that these are really manifestations. I'm getting rid of the three columns, because people are interpreting those as linear, too. Rather, these are manifestations tied in with diversity of pattern. What I'm really saying is that I would expect pragmatic in the least diverse pattern, with imaginative more diverse, and visionary even more diverse. So it's really diversity of pattern and these as being observable manifestations, according to how you might or might not define them.

BJS: If you were looking at a human field that was pragmatic, what kind of characteristics might it have?

MER: Well, there you get into really, in a sense, definition. And I use them, again, in the general language sense, meaning not at all as a psychologist or anybody else would define it. And I think that certainly, until I know more, I don't want to get into greater specificity, because certain definitions taken from other fields are not going to be valid for this. So what I keep trying to say is, unless it has been defined specifically in the glossary, only the general language definition has relevance. And then I'm going to have to buy myself a new dictionary! Sooner or later there is going to have to be more specificity, but these are all the manifestations of field pattern, as stated here. But they tie into both the nature of diversity and the relative nature of diversity. Okay?

BJS: Yes. How does life reconcile mechanical and conscious processes?

MER: I would say it doesn't.

BJS: The reason I ask is that was a statement you had made.

MER: I'm not using "consciousness" in this book, because, again, it has so many, many meanings. You know, a nurse working in the emergency room will write that somebody came in unconscious. But if you get somebody out of Freud, consciousness has an entirely different meaning. And I am trying to avoid all of those terms that have become quite ambiguous.

I think one of the things, now—in relation to the building blocks, or postulates—I'm really talking about basically energy fields, openness, pattern, and four-dimensionality. Now, that's a little different from the original book. When I got into that last chapter on sentience, reason, and feelings, it didn't really fit with the others. I put it in knowing it didn't, but because in talking with different people before, people were getting the idea that this was mechanistic, a bunch of physics. So I wanted to get across the point early that I was talking about people who manifest—or have a little blood running in their veins. What those really are, are manifestation of pattern. It doesn't constitute a basic postulate or assumption at all. So, while I'll be retaining in this new book a lot of that chapter, it's going to be placed differently. It will be dealt with as a manifestation of field, rather than in the other spot. You see, the mechanists really are dealing with parts, so within this system they have no place. Consciousness, no matter whether one is in the ER or sitting in Freud's laboratory, is still a manifestation of field; I see them as two entirely different things. One is a behavior, the other is—well, they both are in that sense—but I don't buy the mechanism for lots of reasons. One, I don't think man is $1.98 worth of chemicals, or a six million dollar man, for that matter; and I don't make any effort to try to explain how these things happened. I just say, "This is what I see, and these are the kinds of things that would explain these." If you want to push it further, you'll have to do it yourself.

BJS: When you said that one of these is a behavior, you meant that consciousness is a behavior?

MER: Yes. It's a manifestation of pattern.

BJS: What is your opinion of the Neo-Darwinian view of evolution?

MER: I don't really feel particularly competent to discuss Neo-Darwinism. I am familiar with it, of course, through some reading, but—certainly as knowledge has increased beyond Darwin's original work, we've learned lots of things. I think Neo-Darwinism is simply an effort to go beyond, using newer knowledge that we have available. I think that, certainly, now in the literature there are proposals that outdistance the Neo-Darwinists by far. So, I think, really it's more a manifestation of growing knowledge or accelerating science and technology. But as far as any scholarly dissertation on it, I wouldn't consider myself competent to do anything.

BJS: How do you account for the orderliness of man's becoming?

MER: I guess some of these things I sort of avoid, because I don't think that life—that evolution—is chaos. At the same time, I'm inclined to think that maybe we're going to find a lot of paradoxes in what we think is order. And some of the things, maybe as we know more, that we think look chaotic, are not chaotic. On the other hand, in a sense, I don't think that it is randomness, in the sense that I think the term is commonly used. Do I think there is purpose or meaning? I wouldn't know. It's a pretty wonderful world we live in, so I'll put it down to my ignorance and say I'll accept things. As we know more, we ought to—I think it's a wonderful world. There is a kind of order in this, but again, I don't think I could define it; and by this I don't mean all the ducks in a row.

BJS: But you are able to derive some correlates and identify some kind of a trend in the patterning.

MER: I don't know what I'll do with that phrase; it's really a very nice one.

BJS: What is the nature, or essential quality, of the human energy field?

MER: What do you mean by "nature or essential quality?"

BJS: I guess where I was coming from there was, the old philosophical idea of some basic quality, or nature, to the universe. The old divisions are matter versus spirit or mind versus matter.

MER: You see, that doesn't fit with this system at all.

BJS: For example, when we talk about the human energy field, what is that energy? It's tied in with, "What is your definition of energy?"

MER: It's just a definition. It's more like "Which came first, the chicken or the egg?" And who's to know? But, certainly definition, I think, is one of the ways that is a good aid to thinking and, certainly, I'm still working to improve that definition of both human field and environmental field. So there may be some minor word changes in that. What I mean won't change, but maybe I'll communicate better.

One starts with the field and gets to the conceptual system; and the conceptual system deals with human and environmental fields, so it's all tied in together. One of the things that I wondered when I heard that question—over the last few years an awful lot of people have been saying, "Well, what is the essence?" The idea, as near as I can figure out being that what they really meant was soul, or spirit, or something like that; which I don't get into, either, because I see man as a human field that manifests all kinds of things. If I were going to say the essence, or nature, I'd have to say, "pattern." I don't know anything to say. But I won't get mixed up with people's commitments to some of these other things, because nobody means the same thing by them, and that's all right with me. They can do whatever they want to it; but I don't think it's something that sits out here and grows on a tree and you pick it off when you want it. Energy I have defined.

BJS: What is the status or role of the gene in the human energy field?

MER: The role of the gene has gone out of style very early. I think it served a good purpose, in the sense of studies and all sorts of things, but it is a part. The other thing is, there is an awful lot of evidence that the genes are not the things that do all of this. The extrachromosomal genetic system has been demonstrated to be just as important as the genetic system; and when one deals with fields, there are no parts, so that it has no status or role in terms of the field.

BJS: Where does personality fit into this scheme?

MER: Person, whatever that is, is a manifestation of pattern. Here, again, personality has taken on all sorts of psychological stereotypes. I'm trying to avoid words that have been heavily associated with the traditional sciences, simply, hopefully, so that I can communicate better. I don't think I will completely, because nobody ever really knows how to put down all the things one is thinking, anyway.

BJS: How does human consciousness develop and manifest?

MER: "Consciousness." Here, again, is a word that I simply don't use and I haven't used in a long time.

BJS: I'll tell you how I'm using it, if that will make any difference—in the sense of "awareness."

MER: Now, the term "awareness" I have used and I probably will continue to use it. It doesn't have all the connotations that "consciousness" has, and I don't think it would create so much misunderstanding. I've used the term "perception" some, but more and more I'm beginning to think it's a bad word to use, because it also is gaining in its jargon, in the sense that it's being used in many different circles. I've discovered in nursing, in some circles, it's becoming almost a fad. Well, when things get that way, then I know I'm going to be in trouble. So I will avoid as much as I can the term "perception," just because I know it's being used in different ways, not because I think it's a bad word. If I do use any of those, then I'm going to have to add a definition; otherwise I'll be in trouble. "Consciousness," I felt, was better just to forget about. But "awareness" I have continued to use, for want of a better word, and I haven't found a better one. I think that I do go along with the writers that propose that consciousness is rudimentary throughout the universe. It's sort of like, how do you differentiate between life and nonlife? But that's a pretty global definition.

BJS: That's how I am using it, definitely.

MER: I think as far as pattern manifesting awareness, it is really a part of this growing diversity. I use "evolution" to mean change. As I get into it, I'm finding that "change" is probably a better word, because there are so many fundamentalists who get all upset at the word "evolution" and then don't hear anything you're saying. So in speeches I've tried to avoid the word, because once in a while I run across somebody who hasn't the remotest idea what I'm talking about, but gets angry with the word "evolution." I am talking more about change, which everybody is agreed on. You know, change is inevitable, so nobody battles over that one much. But it is manifest—I mean any of these behaviors are manifest—in all sorts of ways. Now the correlates of patterning—I'm working on increasing those, there will be a longer list in the book. What's going to happen with those, I'm quite sure, is I'm going to have to write another book after this one. I know I'm not going to have last answers. But I learned a long time ago, you can't wait until you have it all, or you're immobilized. So you do the best you can and you add a P.S. and say, "Look for the next revision. It will be along!"

BJS: If four-dimensionality is neither spatial nor temporal, how can you describe evolution as occuring within space and time? I think this came out of the old unidirectionality assumption.

MER: Yes, and evolution doesn't occur within space and time. I have a whole chapter on four-dimensionality, because that's causing people more confusion than anything else. We've all grown up in a three-dimensional reality with a linear time line, and everything in the real world, whatever we meant, that was a solid. And, of course, there is a perfectly valid spatial fourth dimension as far as that goes, whether one is labeling it supercubes or something else. There's nothing wrong with it, as long as one sees it within that context. It is generated by a solid, and people who work with that—mathematicians—theoretically go into all sorts of dimensions. But it the world we've lived in, all other dimensions were abstractions. The only reality was the third dimension. Now, certainly, I was very much stimulated in my thinking by Einstein, and, of course, he pointed out that he had four coordinates, and he dealt with them as a synthesis and came up with a brand new product, which people still don't really recognize. They still want to talk about space and time, which I don't think is what he meant at all. But maybe he meant something else, too. The thing is, what I mean by four-dimensionality does not derive from spatial or temporal. It looks at all sorts of things. And I think the definition that I have now is very good. Now the problem is to interpret it so anybody else knows what I am talking about, because the language is not replete with such terms. But what I'm saying is that four-dimensionality is where reality is. Certainly, before Euclid got into his spatial geometry, that didn't mean that depth, length, and breadth didn't exist before. He pulled them together and said this is the real world, and it's been around for a few thousand years. What I'm saying is that you can have all this other you want, but it's an abstraction. It has no reality. The only reality is this four-dimensional world; and one can have multiple dimensions if one wants to, but they're not real. I'm saying that the human and environmental fields are four-dimensional. It is a nonlinear domain without spatial or temporal attributes, and when you think of human and environmental fields as integral and infinite, as I've talked about them, then I think maybe it helps to make it clear. Clearer, anyway.

BJS: Can four-dimensionality be correlated with the concepts of consciousness or soul?

MER: I don't think it's a question of being correlated. The principles and theories derive from the totality of the system; they do not derive from any of the building blocks. The system is a synthesis and transcendence. It is a new product. It has its own unity. The system is a synthesis of facts and ideas. But one doesn't study the building blocks; one studies the system. I wouldn't say it isn't correlated with, but it is integral to, the system. I don't really tie up consciousness and soul as being the same thing.

BJS: No. How about awareness? How about if we just crossed all that out and tried to connect awareness to four-dimensionality?

MER: That isn't connectible. Nothing is, because awareness is a manifestation, and consciousness and soul—whatever one means by these—are manifestations of pattern that derive out of the system, not out of any piece of it. I am having a chapter on the conceptual system in which I try to synthesize so that it all has some meaning. Hopefully, then, people will have a better understanding of where some of these attributes, or characteristics, or manifestations, are coming from. I'm trying to avoid the use of the word "behavior" because it's been, again, so associated with biological behavior or psychological behavior that in trying to communicate, it just doesn't seem like a good word.

BJS: If the boundaries of the human energy field are imaginary, are there really no individual units? No wholes?

MER: There are no boundaries, anyway.

BJS: Please explain how your view is humanistic, not mechanistic.

MER: I guess my view is humanistic in the sense that it certainly isn't mechanistic; it doesn't deal with just a machine. Rather, in a general language sense, I think of people as manifesting feelings and reason and those things that we generally associate with being human. Just because I say man manifests certain things, I have not said that nothing else manifests them. That's one of those forms of illogic that a lot of people want to jump from. If you don't mention them, then obviously nothing else does. So I may have to insert a sentence to make it clear that this is not comparative or anything of that sort.

BJS: What is your current view of self-regulation?

MER: It's a static concept; I tried to redefine it. Self-regulation has no place in this system. It derived from a closed-system model, from a static model. I was thinking of Canon as being a major proponent, and, of course, he was dealing with homeostatis—"like static." And, of course, that's been demonstrably outdated for 25 years in the literature. Then we began to get into outer space exploration, and it became evident that things like homeostasis and equilibrium and steady state just were antiquated. So please omit every reference to it.

BJS: How can man be subject to influence not physically at hand?

MER: There are manifestations of field, just as any of those other correlations are manifestations. They are manifestations of the nature and diversity of pattern. At this point we do have evidence that diversity is real, that it is growing. We're beginning to get a little work on the nature of the diversity, but we need a whole lot more. I think these correlates are efforts to get at the nature of the diversity, and I think they'll be helpful. Somebody just left me something she's working on. She's struggling to get to her design. I think she gets into sleep/waking/beyond waking. What we get into there, again, are definitions, because the work done in that area is viewing sleep/waking as either a biological phenomenon or a psychological one, and we're not concerned with those. Rather, how can one look at this as a field phenomenon?

BJS: Does the Indian concept of a hierarchy of energy centers in the human being seem compatible with your paradigm?

MER: These split man up in ways that an irreducible system cannot be split. I am getting further into some of the Eastern philosophies and religions before I finish up. Whether one can deal with some of these things as manifestations of pattern, I don't know. . . . There are similarities in many places.

BJS: Dr. Krieger, in the First National Rogerian Conference, stated that man has an innate coherence and is syntropic—holding a fundamental drive towards order. She also stated that the direction of human evolution is toward infinity. Is this a valid interpretation of your model?

MER: On Dee, basically in most ways we go along together; and, certainly, the work she does is remarkable. I know her therapeutic touch works.

We debate sometimes endlessly on some of the differences we have in terms of theoretical rationale. When one talks about syntropy from a dictionary definition, one is talking about primarily physical patterning. . . .So it really, in a sense, is irrelevant. I think there are lots of things in terms of patterning; and the more work I do in this area, the more important I think pattern is. I think that it's a place where we need to really get into a lot of basic research.

BJS: Please clarify the term "probabilistic purposiveness."

MER: This little phrase, I think, probably came out of my book. "Probabilistic" is going to stay all over the place. "Purposive" probably won't. There are terms that trouble me, like purposiveness, intentionality, and goal-directedness, which I don't buy. I think part of it may be because, in general, they're used in a very pragmatic sense, which I don't think has relevance in a philosophical system. I think that there are many potentialities, and some will be actualized and some won't. But I do not believe that there is any goal that says, "This actuality is going to happen, instead of that." So, to that extent, I'm not at all sure I'll say that in that book. I think it needs a lot more thinking.

BJS: How can there be rhythms but no repetition?

MER: Now, there's nothing that says rhythms have to be repetitions; as a matter of fact, I would say even on an everyday level people are aware that they don't. There's a great deal of recognition that change is inevitable, and if you have inevitable change, then rhythms are nonrepeating. I think that because of this closed-system model of the universe, people have tended to see this as circular. The whole robot world is one of repetition, which is an entirely different level of discourse. I would say that there is no repetition. Certainly, this is supported in Prigogine's work; it's supported in a range of other pieces.

BJS: How do you derive the indices of human development from the trend toward increasing diversity alone?

MER: I've quit using the word "development," because, again, it's ambiguous. People tend to think a lot of psychological, physical, social, biological, or so on; so that it's taken on a stereotype, and it has none of the global meaning for the evolutionary process. So, I'm talking about patterning.

BJS: One more thing that I wanted to ask you about is Cowling's dissertation on mystical experience. Would you see mystical awareness as a manifestation of diversity of pattern?

MER: Yes. Of the nature of the pattern. I perceive in this model again as a developmental process, and dying as a developmental process. Patterning doesn't need a physical body and a physical spectrum in order to persist; I'm not talking about a physical body. So, I would perceive some of the things that Richard was dealing with as manifestations of pattern.

January 31, 1984

BJS: One of the things that I really want to focus on today is, first of all, pattern. In the last interview, you said that pattern was really the basic element of your model.

MER: It is a very key concept. Now, it couldn't exist without all of the other things. I did give you the updated definitions. It is perceived as a single wave. I will not be using the term "pattern" at all in the book, except when it is used to mean exactly how I have defined it. I'm having to be very careful in editing that whole thing, that I use terms in ways that will not be confusing. A system is a synthesis. Pattern and, of course, energy fields, four-dimensionality, and openness are synthesized and are defined so that they are not, per se, subject to study. They're assumed. I postulate these are so. Now, when one gets into pattern's significance in relation to basic research, then, we get at manifestations of pattern, really, which can be quite abstract. The concept of patterning is a general concept. In terms of deriving theories that would deal with the nature of patterning, that's a different kind of query. The reason I'm getting into that is because people apparently have been confused about thinking that they should be studying the building blocks; whereas theories do not derive from the building blocks, they derive from the system. When people haven't seen the idea of deriving from the system, it's gotten them into some trouble, and it's gotten me into some trouble. But pattern is the identifying characteristic.

BJS: So the universe consists of energy fields. And they are infinite. They're integral. And the way we can identify individual energy fields is by their pattern.

MER: It's not how we do it; energy fields *are* identified by their pattern. When we get into trying to identify the nature and direction of change, then we're dealing with manifestations of pattern. It's the identifying characteristic. But we never see pattern in the abstract sense; it's like, you can't see the apple in the seed, but you can imagine it.

BJS: That's interesting that you brought up that idea, because one article I was reading used the word "pattern" and compared it to Aristotle's "form," which is the thing that causes, for example, the seed to grow into an apple. It is the form, or the pattern, inherent in the seed.

MER: But that would be a contradiction of what I am talking about. Somebody wrote, "It's easy to see the seeds in the apple, but it requires imagination to see the apple in the seed." Thank you for your input; I would not want people to see this as Aristotelian, because he was dealing with a closed, causal system. I would have to say that I would disagree with what he said, because the apple isn't inherent in that same sense. Rather, it is a manifestation of the mutual process.

BJS: Would genes also be a manifestation of pattern?

MER: I would say they are parts. So I would have to say, no—which may be tied more to the general literature and the pervasive view, because genes are handled like hearts and circulatory systems. While I would say that everything is a manifestation of the whole in this integral process, the study of genes will not tell us about human beings.

BJS: We're talking about wholes. Now, the field is a whole.

MER: The human field and the environmental field. They are each unique, and they are unique to each other. My environmental field is different from yours.

BJS: And your human field is different from mine; it's a whole in itself. Even though it's integral and infinite, it's still a whole.

MER: It is irreducible. A friend sent me four books. She is a Buddhist and thought there were similarities and thought I would be interested, which of course I was.

BJS: Yes, some ancient Indian philosophies—

MER: They all have major similarities. Certainly they have a sense of integralness, I think, that transcends the Western view.

BJS: Are pattern and holism related?

MER: Pattern is that which identifies the whole. They're not the same thing. I'm trying to think of some analogy. You know those pictures that children draw, the animals they find in the dots? Now, that's a pattern. But a child would say, "There's a dog." It's a pattern that the child perceives, but pattern is not the dog. Or the old saga about the pile of stones. If you see a wall, it's the pattern that you perceive as the wall. Not the stones. They're not the same thing. The whole is itself, is this irreducible energy field that is infinite. Pattern is that which gives it identity. But you could have a whole even before anybody dreamed up the idea that it was pattern that identified it.

BJS: If you are looking at a human being, would you say "That is a pattern," or would you say "It is identified by pattern"?

MER: If I'm talking about this unitary human being, the physical body isn't a human being. We perceive our own limitations, I guess, maybe more than anything else. . .Here's something I was rewriting to see if it would make better sense. This, at least, is the most recent readable stuff, anyway.

BJS: "Evolution of unitary human beings." So you are still going to use the word "evolution." You were thinking of not using that word.

MER: Well, you know, I'm starting to think about the old allegory about the man, his donkey, and the wood. . . . A perfectly good word should not be thrown out just because somebody doesn't like it; because no matter what else you choose, somebody's not going to like that either. And "evolution" is a perfectly good word. It means change; it means evolving. You can't please everybody. So I will use it—with care, but I will use it.

BJS: Now, most of the definitions of evolution that I've come across specify that evolution is change in some sort of a direction, where there is some continuity.

MER: I use it as the dictionary defines it, in the general sense. I'm sure we're both aware where the battle lies—in fundamentalists who want to deny evolutionary theory as opposed to some other belief, change versus stasis, and so on. And I had thought maybe to get around it. But maybe there are some things that one shouldn't even bother with trying to get around. All terms are defined in the general language sense, unless they are defined specifically by me in the context of in the glossary. And I hope that people will have a dictionary. I'll check mine out against the large dictionary. I am checking them out against the college dictionaries, because those are the ones that people are apt to go to. They're not so bad.

BJS: Increasing diversity is another thing I wanted to ask you about. These are manifestations of relative diversity in field patterning [quoting from handout] "from lesser diversity to greater diversity, longer rhythms to shorter rhythms." And the rhythmicity is where the word "wave" comes from? That's the sense in which you were using wave?

MER: Yes. The minute you have any kind of a column, people tend to want to make it all linear. That is not the intent. Also, these are relative to the individual. The change is not from here to here. I am told that there are people who do interpret it that way. I hear these things and I try to find out what kinds of confusion I've put people into. To that extent, I'll try to do something about it.

BJS: Now, the pragmatic to the visionary, and materiality to ethereal—these all seem to be four-dimensional.

MER: I know; they are not. Here is one of the big holes that people are falling into. People do not move into four-dimensionality. Reality is four-dimensional, and if it is true, it was here long before I or anybody else recognized it. It's part of these building blocks. So any person is just as much four-dimensional, even though he may have manifestations of patterning of far less diversity. He's just as four-dimensional as somebody over here. I'm finding that a good many people have been interpreting it the other way, and I can understand how it happened, because four-dimensionality has become—with all the interest in paranormal and other sorts of things—sort of an "in" idea right now. Whether or not I contributed to the confusion—it's quite possible I did, I don't know—I'm going to try to undo it.

BJS: People think of it as some sort of an experience—"I'm going to have this experience of four-dimensionality." But it's the condition of our existence, right? I mean, reality is four-dimensional, we are four-dimensional. If we are looking at the world through three-dimensional spectacles, that still doesn't mean that we are not four-dimensional.

MER: When Euclid pulled together all sorts of things about spatial geometry, he set up Euclidean spatial geometry, with a linear time line. And whatever the world is, it's been like that. He just simply drew a picture of what he thought reality was like, and it's served us rather well for a few thousand years. Now, it didn't mean that it was any more true than something else. It didn't throw out other dimensions; it said they were all abstract. But everything in the real world that we've been living with, as far as we were concerned, had been three-dimensional. Now, actually, that began to change when Einstein threw in relativity; but nobody knew what he was talking about then. So, as time has gone on, it's come to the point where people are talking about four-dimensionality all over the place. We see it a lot in books and various sorts of things. Certainly, it isn't the first time other dimensions were talked about. I really got caught the other day; a biblical scholar reminded me that in Revelation, in the New Testament, they talk about more dimensions. I'm going back to reread that, but it seems to me they talked about seven. So, again, the thing here is, it has been defined and it is simply saying that, "If you want a three-dimensional world you can have it; but it's an abstraction; it has no reality. The only reality is four-dimensional."

BJS: You say four-dimensionality is a nonlinear, nonspatial, nontemporal domain. Can you describe it in any positive terms, rather than what it isn't?

MER: Those are positive terms in the sense that "entropy" was the "in" word, and when they began to recognize that maybe things weren't so closed, they said "negative entropy." What they were saying, in that particular instance, was, it was the "opposite form." Well, so with nonspatial and nontemporal, there's nothing really negative about them. It is a very positive description—in words that are at least in the dictionary. Frankly, I feel pretty good about it. I think it's another thing to try to describe. I have been collecting different things from the literature, like a phrase or something. I think "Aha!" I will not use them as such, but they seem to give me some ideas about how I can improve my explanations. Now, I must say, that chapter has given me a fair amount of trouble. It will not be a long one.

BJS: What phrases have you come across? Can you remember any of them?

MER: No. They stimulate an "aha," but the "aha" may bear no relationship to what it was. That kind of thing, sort of thinking, "now that gives me an idea." It transcends the coordinates, and my hunch is that is what Einstein was doing, although I don't think he was necessarily talking about the same thing I am. But he was talking about synthesizing, and when you synthesize you transcend, you come up with a new product that is irreducible. And he was saying, "It's only one word; it isn't these things." These things don't make it; it isn't something you add. He didn't derive his concept from a spatial system. What I mean by four-dimensionality in this cannot be bound by spatial geometry, at all. Now, nontemporal has been a concept that has been held by theoretical physicists for a century. More recently, they made it quite clear that there is no such thing as universal time. Certainly that was true when they began to play around with quantum theory. I perceive the definition as being a positive statement of what it is, rather than what it isn't. Nonlinearity is very much part of our language today, whether one is talking about the so-called basic sciences, or math, or stat, or all these other areas. What it's saying is it spreads all over, it's not a line. It does represent a transcendence. Now there's some discussion of that in here [the book on Buddhism]. And when people talk about some of these areas in the literature, they do talk about transcendence. Nobody's proposed language that *would*—although I think there certainly are people who obviously are perceiving a domain that is infinite. You see, we've been so long in this spatial orientation, that there is a great desire to say, "Expands in directions we don't know about." But it can't, not in a nonspatial definition. It is abstract, and I think that it's harder to see than the apple in the seed. Some of that's because we are not accustomed to thinking in terms of a four-dimensional reality, whereas apples we have all over the place. But I think the analogy is good.

BJS: One of the things I wanted to ask you about again was "pragmatic" and "visionary," because I looked these words up in the dictionary.

MER: Pragmatic, imaginative, and visionary—I've been using them for a long time. They represent increasing diversity, relatively, with higher-frequency field patterning.

BJS: You're not speaking of those as mental states or anything. I ask because the dictionary definitions leaned toward that. Imagination it defined as "able to form mental images," but I knew you weren't talking about that.

MER: It is either a dichotomized or particulate or analytic view of the world which gets them into the dictionary, whereas these are field manifestations. Sleeping/waking/beyond waking is just as ambiguous, because the work that's been done has pretty much been either biological or psychological.

BJS: Right. And you are not talking about that.

MER: I'm not talking about sleep as a biological phenomenon or a psychological one. I have wanted to avoid a long glossary, and I've been trying to do it on the basis of pointing out that all behaviors, characteristics, attributes—whatever you label them—are field manifestations. They're not dealt with as manifestations of a part or anything of that sort. Whether or not the message will get across, I don't know; but I think that I would be in a bad way if I got started trying to define everything. It just wouldn't work. Now, we'll be discussing these (correlates) in detail.

BJS: What about materiality and ethereal? What do you want to do with them?

MER: I don't know what I'm going to do with them. I may change the word. What we get into is, in a pragmatic sense, people tend to think it's about mass versus—the other. And what I'm trying to get at here is it's really perception, I guess, although I've got some better words for that. I won't be using "perception." We did some looking in the dictionary, and "conception" is a much better word, or "experienced as."

BJS: Oh, I see, I see.

MER: So I won't be using "perception" at all. I like "experienced as" the best, because I think it's a more global sort of thing. We get into the traditional business of everybody thinking that we learn about our world with the five senses, despite Einstein's statement of mass as the same as energy. This has been looked at by people in the lines of fields, and Polanyi has talked about it; nonetheless, the man in the street doesn't, and neither does the nurse or much of anybody else. The materiality is really matter—and it's that word, I think, which is a poor choice. Whereas, "ethereal" poets use it, or somebody says "they're so fragile I thought I could see right through them." In other words, "experienced as ethereal." The visible spectrum—it's very little that we perceive. We know that there are people who can experience infrared, ultraviolet, etc. People who deal with colors are in the process of saying that the visible spectrum just isn't any good anymore, because they now perceive so many shades. If you get color charts, they'll be big things. If you look at all they have laid out—relationships, you know—many people will not differentiate. Well, there was a time, at least if one believes in the literature, when black and white were the only things perceived. There were no colors.

BJS: That's interesting, because infants can only perceive black and white.

MER: That's what they're saying. They may be right. I don't think it's as simple as they're saying. One should keep an open mind. There's no question that it's changing very rapidly, in all of these areas. It may very well provide a tool in terms of infants' pattern and diversity and relative differencs, more diverse patterning in infants, those would perceive differently or experience things differently from the less diverse. And then we'd have the Smiths trying to be like the Joneses. I'd like to do away with the old hierarchical view, to perceive the individual not as somebody better than or less than. Now, whether or not that's possible, I don't know. People seem to like a hierarchy.

BJS: That's true. Most of the evolutionary philosophers that I've been reading really like to create their hierarchies.

MER: I think it's all pretty heavily value-laden; of course it's very integral to cultures—not to all cultures, apparently. At any rate, when you get into a non-linear domain, then you're also getting away from hierarchical structures. One can have difference and diversity without having a hierarchy.

BJS: Would you still put any value on ideas like species, and things like that—meaning groups of fields that have similar patterning?

MER: No, I stay clear away from it, for a lot of reasons. The purpose of this model is to look at people. It doesn't make them better or less or anything else. I think the uniqueness and diversity of the life and nonlife on this planet is incredible. I don't think one is better or less than another. My concern is with people. Now I think, certainly, one can learn many things. The more one knows, the more ideas one gets. But I do not see including that, in terms of what I'm writing, or comparative things.

BJS: So you wouldn't say that human beings, as a group, are more diverse than other forms of life?

MER: No.

BJS: So it's just that for an individual human being, evolution is toward greater diversity.

MER: Of his own pattern. You know, we get into some very interesting things. People keep talking about how higher apes can't talk English. Well, I haven't noticed any Englishmen talking ape language either. In other words, I think we have to value differences and stop thinking that if it isn't like us, it can't be as good so that it's, rather, to value differences, to respect them, and, as a matter of fact, enjoy them. I think it is in this overwhelming diversity that the planet is so wonderful—not in man's sitting up on a peak. There are people still around who want to say that man isn't another animal at all. You've got man, and then a gap, and then here are the animals.

BJS: In the master's curriculum there's a course that's called Evolutionary Emergence. Does that concept fit, at all, into what you're talking about?

MER: Well, I can't tell you what's going on in that class right now, but in terms of evolutionary emergence, the universe is continually changing, evolving. Whatever it is, it's becoming more diverse. There is no repetition. And that's been, after all, what Prigogine got a Nobel Prize for pointing out. Now, historically the idea—well, Darwin started his—of course, all hell broke loose because man was supposed to come from the ape. People drew pictures and still have them all over the place, and they are still trying to see where man broke off from the apes. Well, I don't know whether, what man, where—we've got big gaps in our knowledge. And we also have gaps in our capacity to interpret what we do see. So I think that evolution, or change, is vastly more complex and exciting than any straight-line branching. Now, it doesn't bother me a bit if way, way back there, apes preceded; something preceded. It was one whale of a long time ago, because we can go back thousands and thousands and thousands of years and still identify something we call human. Some of these other animals have bigger brain cages than man. It isn't the size of the brain that determines. Now, one can argue, microcephalic, but one doesn't have to get involved in deformities. But it is field pattern that determines. So in a period of accelerating change, we are able to see more directly this growing diversity. When we were thinking in terms of a thousand, ten thousand years, it didn't seem like change was happening. Now, I think we are on the threshold of outer space, and I think we can expect even moe marked changes and diversity in the future. We couldn't even imagine them in the past. What this will mean, I don't know. It's anybody's guess. So I will not be dealing with any comparaive anatomy. The other thing is with the idea of fields, anatomy becomes irrelevant.

BJS: I know you say that patterning continues beyond death—what we call death.

MER: I talk about dying. What I say is that field patterning is continuous, and is not determined by something called death or nondeath, or by living or nonliving. If energy fields are the fundamental unit of the universe, then all fields are identified pattern. Now, the selection of a field for study is arbitrary. Cell physiologists have studied cells as fields. That's all right. It depends on who's doing what. The identification of any particular field is arbitrary. It's false, in the sense that fields are infinite; a field is infinite, but there's nothing wrong about it.

BJS: What about our sense of self? Most people have a sense of self, that they are some sort of an enduring—

MER: I guess that's a good thing to have. It's a field manifestation. And the nature of it is unique to each individual. You better read some of this [on Buddhism]. It's amazing. This goes back so long and yet discusses, from a historical Buddhist perception, exactly what you're talking about.

BJS: Oh yes, mystical experience. One of the first things to go is the sense of self. And I know it's considered to be an illusion by many of the Eastern philosophies.

MER: Well, I believe in ego! [laughing]

BJS: Now, I know that we're a universe of open systems, and open systems are negentropic.

MER: Entropy is based on a closed-system model. It was introduced in physics, and everything was to be running down. Negative entropy was the way it started—in negative entropy you have open systems with everything getting more complex, diverse, heterogeneous, not running down.

BJS: Right. So then when you say pattern is becoming more diverse, why do you not say it is becoming more complex and heterogenous and differentiated? Wouldn't it be, since it's open systems?

MER: To get away from confusion and ambiguity. I decided one word would be much more effective, and it seemed to me that "diversity" would be least misunderstood. It's amazing how people attach different meanings to words. "Complex" was one that really messed people up. They wanted it to be concrete. These other words tended to be stereotyped as things. And so it was, simply, in the hopes that what I was trying to say might come across clearer.

BJS: But it's not that you don't think that fields are becoming more complex and heterogeneous and differentiated.

MER: There are slight differences in meaning of all those words. There was a time when I would talk about all of them, simply hoping that maybe one would get through. But one thing keep in mind. Just because someone has said something is so, he has not said one word about what isn't. In other words, this doesn't mean anything about what isn't. I haven't said what isn't. I haven't said they were heterogeneous or homogeneous in the sense of there's no contradiction. Now, you can't have a more diverse field and have it homogeneous. Of course, it's more heterogeneous. But the real reason was to stick to one word that, hopefully, would be less confusing. I'm struggling a lot with trying to look at the picayune, which drives me up a tree; but I think it's terribly important.

BJS: I wanted to go back to something you said last time, that you agree with those who believe that consciousness is rudimentary throughout the universe—consciousness, in a very broad sense.

MER: Yes. Now, that's another word that I avoid using.

BJS: You prefer to use the word "awareness."

MER: I will not use the word "consciousness" at all.

BJS: So that, maybe, awareness is rudimentary throughout the universe, or some sort of perception?

MER: In those introductory chapters when I was trying to give an overview, I did make some statement that many believe this is so. In terms of historical background, I'll leave it the way people have said it. I will not get into battles with, do plants think or not? What do we mean by the terms? Then, it would get into definitions of specificity. So, it will be, what are man's capacities, not whether these are like or different from. Certainly, there are plants that behave in ways that are similar to what we label consciousness in people. I'm talking about, what are man's potentials? The fact that there may be other things with similar potentials is great. There are. But that doesn't happen to be the primary concern of nursing.

BJS: Many people feel that anything that has some wholeness or unity or integrity or pattern to it has some minimal awareness and that's the only way it can maintain its integrity or wholeness.

MER: You see, they want to throw in causality. Wholeness, if you're dealing with energy fields, is a given. One might not like what one has perceived, but it's a given. Everybody is a whole within his own thing, the nature of which varies. What gets manifest is something else. But I know what you're saying. It's because they're not perceiving a whole as an energy field and they're also trying to add up parts, I suspect. That is one of the problems that people have, generally.

BJS: Pattern is also four-dimensional, right? It's not the idea of pattern as something that's—

MER: Pattern isn't—the world, the universe, these energy fields, are four-dimensional, and pattern identifies this field. Now, certainly, if you look at patterning, particularly in the last 30 or 40 years, there's been a fair amount of concern with patterning in terms people looking at all life, nonlife. I'm saying that patterning—the field, reality—is four-dimensional. Here we're back at what I was saying before. The conceptual system, reality, is a new product. It transcends all these things that went into it. They are synthesized—the field, four-dimensionality, pattern—and there is this irreducible system. You can't deal with reality at all that isn't four-dimensionality, energy fields, identified as pattern.

BJS: I wanted to ask you about David Bohm's *Wholeness and the Implicate Order.* Does that have any connection or relevance?

MER: I think it's a fascinating book, and he's done some other fascinating ones, too, although that's really the most recent. I would say he's much closer to the kind of things I'm talking about, than, say, he was in some of his earlier things. There are points when I see something familiar. But, no; we are not talking about the same thing, in that the model I have, I think, makes a lot better sense. Part of it is that I was freer to move out of vertical holes. And he's still trying to work it within, essentially, the traditional worldview. As I say, I found his work fascinating. But he doesn't have this.

BJS: So his implicate order isn't really your four-dimensional, nonlinear, nontemporal domain.

MER: No. He isn't calling it that.

BJS: Now, man and the universe are integral. Does that mean that the whole is immanent in every field? Hegel called the whole the Absolute, and put boundaries around it and it was a closed system. But he said that the whole was immanent in each—

MER: As a matter of fact, you can find in the literature, particularly of philosophers, for a long time, the idea of man being a part of the world. Now, of course, when I say going back a long time, I have to clarify what I mean. In the evolution of life, historically and with a closed-system model, man has seen himself and the environment at odds with one another. But one can find sentences or paragraphs in different places where the "man at one with nature" theme does appear, particularly in literary kinds of things. So that, itself, is not unusual. But it is still talking about man as a physical body, in a three-dimensional universe, essentially static, as well as closed. I think here, again, people can use the same words, but what they mean is something else. You know, the ancient Greeks talked about atoms, but they sure weren't talking about what somebody today means by an atom. I don't know if we'll ever get out of the morass of words. That Tower of Babel ought to be around now. I think with any one of those, one has to read within the total context.

BJS: Mainly, I was really wanting to zero in on pattern, wholeness, four-dimensionality, and the direction of change.

MER: Most of them are defined as givens. The direction of change is tied in with the principles of homeodynamics, which get at the nature and direction of change. Here, I'm having to be very, very careful, because direction, to most people, tends to mean linearity, which is not what I mean, but rather, growing diversity of field pattern. And it's probabilistic and continuous, so there is no direction in the pervasive meaning of that term.

BJS: It's probabilistic, meaning it can be predicted somewhat?

MER: Probability says you can't know—the principle of uncertainty. There are many potentialities; only some will be actualized. Whatever is actualized is going to be novel, new, innovative, creative. But there's no way of predicting. Now, we do make probabilistic predictions. But we can only do that on large numbers. To predict for the individual is fallacious. Now, that doesn't mean that, in a pragmatic sense, we can't make knowledgeable guesses.

BJS: That's what the correlates are, right?

MER: Right. Yes. But these stand for more diverse manifestations. Where there's unending rhythmicity so that there's always innovation, we get clues. But whatever we see is going to be completely new.